HEALTH REGULATION

Certificate of Need and 1122

Contributors

Robert M. Crane, M.B.A.
Chief, Regulatory Methods Branch
Division of Regulatory Activities
Bureau of Health Planning and
   Resources Development
Health Resources Administration, HEW
5600 Fishers Lane
Rockville, Maryland 20852

Edward J. Hanley, B.A.
Vice-President
Lewin and Associates
Suite 4100
470 L'Enfant Plaza East, S.W.
Washington, D.C. 20024

Leonard H. Glantz, J.D.
Staff Attorney
Center for Law and Health Sciences
Boston U. School of Law
209 Bay State Road
Boston, Massachusetts 02215

Dr. Carolyn Harmon, Ph.D.
Senior Consultant
Lewin and Associates
Suite 4100
470 L'Enfant Plaza East, S.W.
Washington, D.C. 20024

Clayton Medeiros, M.U.P.
(Master's Degree in Urban Planning)
Regional Consultant for Health Planning
Division of Resources and Development
Public Health Service, Room 3300
Regional Office
26 Federal Plaza
New York, New York 10007

HEALTH REGULATION

Certificate of Need and 1122

Herbert Harvey Hyman, Ph. D.

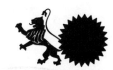

Aspen Systems Corporation
Germantown, Maryland
1977

"This publication is designed to provide accurate
and authoritative information in regard to the
Subject Matter covered. It is sold with the
understanding that the publisher is not engaged in
rendering legal, accounting, or other professional
service. If legal advice or other expert assistance is
required, the services of a competent professional
person should be sought." From a Declaration of
Principles jointly adopted by a Committee of the
American Bar Association and a Committee
of Publishers and Associations.

Library of Congress Catalog Card Number: 76-455-24
ISBN: 0-912862-34-3

Printed in the United States of America

2 3 4 5

Table of Contents

Preface

With the passage of the National Health Planning and Resources Development Act of 1974 (PL 93-641), a new chapter in health planning and health regulation has been opened. Many of the concepts that have been discussed for many years in the health planning and health care field have been explicitly articulated in the new law. Among these concepts are the systems approach to planning, the linkage between planning and regulation, and the regional, integrated approach to health care.

One of the major changes that has occurred is the mandatory requirement that every state develop a Certificate of Need program by 1980. This requirement calls for minimum criteria and procedures that every state and the HSAs within these states must meet. These minimum requirements go beyond those that have existed in most states. Health providers should be aware of such requirements and their impact. It requires carefully articulated goals, a clear specification of the target population of its proposal, and how it meets the goals and priorities of the region's long range health goals among others.

In addition, the Act is explicit in linking new institutional facilities and services to the planning goals of the region and the state. This will have a major impact on health providers, because they now must be aware that the needs of their institutions are no longer viewed in the context of what benefits only their patients. Rather, needs will be evaluated from the perspective of the region as a whole and the needs of its population.

The new law also promotes a major shift in how change occurs in a region. The Health Systems Agencies (HSAs), unlike the predecessor Comprehensive Health Planning Agencies (CHPAs), are expected to take the initiative in determining the health care needs of the region. The health providers in turn will be called upon to respond to the HSAs' long and short range plans by proposing programs to meet those objectives. In the past, it was the other way around. The health provider proposed plans and the CHPA reacted.

These are only three of the major ways PL 93-641 will impact on health planning agencies and health care providers. This volume is written in the context of PL 93-641 to assist the health providers by clarifying what they should know about health regulation and the law and what is expected of them under its Certificate of Need and "1122" provisions. This book further explains the methods that can be used to develop institutional and/or regional plans and the respective advantages and disadvantages of each method. It identifies potential areas of legal challenge that health providers have brought in the past and can bring in the future against health planning agencies developed under PL 93-641. It also clarifies the technical and ethical accountability of health planning agencies and health providers under PL 93-641. Finally, it sets forth implications of the law for achieving the cost containment policy of the Act and ways in which health planning agencies and health providers can more likely accomplish their respective aims.

While PL 93-641 is very complex, this book and its contributing authors aim to inform and shed light on the meaning of the health regulatory sections of the Act with special reference to Certificate of Need and "1122".

Herbert H. Hyman
November 1976

Chapter 1

Introduction to Key Issues in Regulation of Health Facilities and Services

Herbert H. Hyman

This chapter was written by Herbert H. Hyman in his private capacity. No official support or endorsement by the Health Resources Administration of HEW is intended or should be inferred.

"Health: United States 1975," an official HEW publication of information on the cost and provision of medical services, points out that the cost of medical care has been rising faster than the Consumer Price Index.[1] In 1975 the total medical care bill passed the one hundred billion dollar mark for the first time. The greater part of this increase—approximately 40% of the total medical care bill—is attributed to the cost of hospital care and other medical services and is evidenced by the increased cost of a semiprivate room from $30.3 per day in 1950 to $182.1 in 1973.

Over half of this increase has occurred in the past ten years[2] and has caused the public to motivate municipal, state and congressional legislators to question the rapid escalation of medical care and to seek solutions. What is interesting in this rapid escalation is its relationship to federal initiatives to solve medical problems. For example, the shortage of hospital beds after World War II resulted in the passage of the Hill-Burton Act in 1946. The shortage of physicians and allied health professionals has resulted in the passage of legislation to foster growth in medical manpower. The concern with lack of knowledge to eradicate or reduce the causes of diseases responsible for high mortality rates has led to the establishment of the National Institutes of Health (NIH) and its proliferation of funds for medical research, particularly in the biomedical sciences. In the course of solving these and other important medical problems, unanticipated problems were created. The Hill-Burton Act has led to an oversupply and uneven allocation of hospital facilities and

1

beds; the Health Professions Educational Assistance Act has produced an oversupply of certain types of medical practitioners and their uneven geographic distribution in urban areas and in the eastern part of the United States; the development of NIH has led to the development of expensive, specialized equipment which has raised the cost of treating the principle "killers" of our population; and the passage of Titles 18 and 19 of the Social Security Act has substantially increased the access of medical care to the poor and elderly in the last ten years and is mainly responsible for the escalation of medical care costs in the mid-1960s. These four programs have been so successful that one of the unanticipated consequences has been the rapid growth and use of ever more sophisticated and costly medical care services. It was not until the Nixon administration that questions began to be raised about the role the federal government itself played in the rising cost of medical care. As a result of this self-examination, federal health policy makers have questioned the continuation of these successful federal programs and raised the issue of alternative methods of providing effective medical care at lower cost.

Because hospital costs represent the largest share of the nat'on's health costs, this area has received the greatest focus. Additionally, the federal government has found itself more heavily involved in the payments of hospital costs since the passage of Titles 18 and 19 of the Social Security Act. It has been estimated that public payments of hospital care amount to 40% of the total medical bill with the larger share belonging to the federal government. Thus, it is not surprising that the emphasis of federal policy has been on seeking ways to inhibit the growth of hospital costs, identifying more economical ways of providing quality care. This has led to new federal initiatives. The major areas of concern have been the development of Health Maintenance Organizations (HMOs), the use of lower-cost allied health professionals and physician extenders for providing medical care, the development of utilization standards to reduce unnecessary care, and the regulation of the entry of new medical facilities or the expansion of existing facilities and services through the prior determination of need for those services. It is with the latter that this book is concerned because it is in the area of health planning and regulation that policy makers believe exists the greatest potential for controlling the costs of medical care.

The two major works on the subject of hospital regulations have been *Hospital Regulation* by Anne Somers[3] and *Regulating Health Facilities Construction* by Clark Havighurst.[4] Both are excellent works that present in-depth analyses of the extent, implications, and theoretical aspects of health regulation. They come to grips with such issues as how regulation works, why it is needed, and its constitutionality. Perhaps because of the complex nature of the subject, neither author came to any strong conclusions as to what should be done about regulating the medical care field. While this book will consider some of the issues raised in the aforementioned works, it begins with the assumption that the medical care field will have to live with conditions of increasing state and federal regulations. Consequently, this book will cover (1) an analysis of the impact of the regulations supported at the state level through Certificate of Need (CON) legislation and at the federal level by the passage of the Section "1122" amendments to the Social Security Act and (2) the implications of PL 93-641 as it effects the medical community. PL 93-641 appears to fulfill the predictions offered by Somers and Havighurst regarding increased federal and state regulation. The discussion of PL 93-641 as it relates to regulation will include both its impact on and the expectations of the health provider.

Regulations have generally been applied in an industry where (1) the public interest may be affected by that industry and (2) where there is a strong potential that the industry through its monopolistic or collusive actions may adversely affect the public interest.[5] The aim of the regulation is to insure that all persons in the community have access to the services provided by the industry without undue discrimination and at a price they can afford and still provide a reasonable return to the industry.

With respect to medical facilities and the services provided by them, hospitals in many small suburban and rural communities frequently represent a monopoly. On the other hand, in larger urban areas, there are usually several hospitals and other alternative medical facilities to which residents could go for treatment. However, while alternative choices are available, entry to the hospital of a person's choice is still very much limited. The patient's physician usually decides where the patient goes and this is often determined by the physician's affiliation with a medical facility. Further, the patient must have the financial means to pay for the medical care, and a bed must be available at the time the request is made. Any one, or a combination of these factors can drastically limit the patient's choice even in an urban area with a multitude of medical facilities potentially available. These factors have led health regulators to treat medical facilities as though they were monopolistic, whether they are in fact or not. There is no question that the hospital industry has direct consequences on the lives of the people who use and need such services. The hospital industry can greatly benefit or harm those whom it serves or fails to serve. It is for these reasons that Drake believes the hospital industry and medical providers require some form of regulation.[6]

The early attempts at controlling the health industry were through voluntary self-regulation. Section 318 of the Public Health Act of 1964 provided federal funds for assisting in the area-wide planning of health related facilities. The aim was to foster voluntary coordination and cooperation among the hospitals in a region through collaborative planning based on data analysis and allocation of facilities and services according to public need. Some planning was done, much data were collected, but improved coordination in the allocation of resources was not achieved. The area-wide health planning facilities councils were understaffed—usually not more than one or two professionals per council—and had too little authority or moral persuasive power. The councils served as little more than private clubs where agreements could be made for supporting each other's projects. Cost containment and efficiency in the allocation of medical facilities and services were not the real concerns of these planning councils.

Two additional efforts at regional health planning, both voluntary, took place shortly thereafter. The Regional Medical Program (RMP), passed in 1966, was aimed at creating regional networks of delivery systems to deal more effectively with the primary causes of mortality in the United States, i.e., heart disease, cancer, and stroke. A complementary law, the Partnership for Health Act of 1966, was broader based in its area-wide planning intent in that it was to include planning for health facilities as well as for services, physical and mental health, and environmental protection, and planning was to involve the consumer as well as the medical provider and public officials concerned with health matters. Both of these wide-ranging laws were predicated on the voluntary involvement of the participants. The RMP had substantial dollars to offer potential applicants interested in demonstrating and implementing new forms of health delivery systems related to the major disease categories. The Partnership for Health Act had little more than good will and moral suasion to encourage the development and eventual implementation of planning for the region. However, the Partnership for Health Act had insufficient funding to carry out the planning required.

The RMP spent most of its dollars for individual projects without the benefit of region-wide plans to guide the use of those funds. While many positive results were achieved by the RMP, they were more the end product of the creativity of the institutions involved in the projects than of rational forethought on the part of the RMP. In spite of the great efforts and expenditures of funds, neither of these three major voluntary efforts achieved the goal of developing a rationally organized, regional health plan for the allocation of resources to serve the public need. These three acts instead served to maintain the status quo of the health providers while enhancing their prestige. The acts provided no penalties or minimal incentives, and contained no implied threats for failing to develop plans for the effective coordination of medical services.

CERTIFICATES OF NEED

As noted above, whereas voluntarism in its several significant legislative forms did not work, it was the work of health economists who made the major contributions that brought the Certificate of Need (CON) laws into existence. These economists identified the presence of economic factors that prevented the usual market mechanism from achieving cost stabilization, i.e., increasing competition, reduction of customers in periods of inflation and rising prices, and oversupply of services in relation to demand.[7] The most important of these factors in fostering price rises was the role played by the third-party insurance mechanism. This mechanism insulates the patient from directly experiencing the full financial burden of medical expenses. Because of the patient's dependence on his physician for medical treatment, he/she does not usually have freedom of choice in identifying and using alternative methods of treatment, nor is there any economic incentive for the patient to want to have such choices. The physician can usually demand and have the medical facility provide any service or equipment he considers necessary for the patient's care without consideration of the costs involved. Regardless of the medical facility's occupancy rate or the cost of the latest available technology or specialized services, the costs of operating the institution are met by charges to the third-party insurors. Lower occupancy rates usually merit high per diem rates since the same costs are spread among fewer patients. Third-party insurors usually have had little choice except to meet these demands, usually through annual increases in their insurance premiums, because of the public benefit associated with medical care. All of these individual behaviors by consumers, physicians, hospitals, and third-party insurors add up to a collective pattern that is contrary to the way the normal economic mechanism operates under conditions of competition and in response to the laws of supply and demand. The consequence is that market forces do not work in the health field to inhibit the use of medical services or their costs. It is for this reason that one writer concluded that "many students of the industry predict that some form of nonmarket constraints must eventually be imposed."[8]

Hospital administrators have been particularly troubled by this economic cycle of events. In a survey conducted among hospital administrators in 1970, Whiting found that (1) the overwhelming number of administrators believed that they should provide leadership to the community for planning the services needed in the area, (2) the majority disagreed that hospital facilities should be regulated or treated as public utilities, (3) almost 80% agreed that hospitals should submit a certificate of need before being permitted to expand any service or facility and (4) almost 70% felt that the comprehensive health planning agency should have the authority to enforce the plans it developed.[9] Whiting concluded on the basis of his findings that "Minnesota hospital chief executive officers can accept involvement in a planning society, but are most resistant to an externally planned society."[10] The important conclusion drawn from this survey and other research findings is that too many economic factors are at work which prevent the market forces from controlling costs in the health field. It becomes obvious, then, that some outside force is required to effect cost controls. Among the medical providers, the hospital administrators perceive themselves as the qualified leaders to confront the problem of cost containment. For reasons that will be explained, they are most inclined to accept some form of CON process rather than alternative cost control mechanisms. These hospital administrators recognize the necessity of linking CON to an area-wide health plan for which they can provide leadership.

However, having said this, one only has to examine the trend and diversity of CON laws in the states and note the slowness with which states have enacted such legislation. New York was the pioneer state, establishing its CON in 1964. This law has become a model for the nation, yet it was four years before Rhode Island, another pioneer state in health matters, passed its law in 1968 and two more years before California passed its law. Thus, even though the forces at work were strong, especially after the passage of Titles 18 and 19 of the Social Security Act, only three states had passed such laws by 1970. However, in the next three years, a rush of twenty more states passed such laws, including Minnesota.

Why this sudden proliferation of interest in the passage of such laws? One of the reasons is that the New York experience showed that such legislation was not detrimental to the legitimate interests of the medical providers. It tended to bring some order out of the multiplicity of demands made by the providers themselselves for expansion of services and facilities. Not only did the hospital providers not feel the law a threat, but possessing a CON often was a positive inducement permitting providers access to low interest loans and federal grants. A second incentive was the growing concern of congressional leaders and the executive branch over the rapid rise in medical costs. The threat of federal controls motivated many states to enact CON laws to ward off the possibility of more rigid federal regulations. Congress eventually added Section 1122 of PL

93-603, the Social Security Amendments of 1972, as a spur to those states that had not passed CON laws. Two years after the passage of the "1122" amendments, 37 states had opted to establish a state-designated agency for the purpose of implementing the federal law. While the state can revoke an institution's license for violation of its CON laws, the main section of the "1122" amendments is the withholding of that portion of the daily rate paid by Titles 5, 18, and 19 funds of the Social Security Act related to the institution's capital expenditures. PL 93-603 was perceived as a threat of still more severe constraints if the combination of state and federal laws failed to retard the costs of medical care.

A third and often overlooked reason for the proliferation of state CON laws and implementation of "1122" amendments is the secondary goal of granting the comprehensive health planning agencies greater authority in bringing rationality to the provisions and allocation of services. By being involved in the first stage of review for CON, the comprehensive Health Planning Agencies were in a position to make decisions based on criteria, standards, and/or plans they developed for their areas. In this way, not only could duplication of services be avoided and the reduction of costs brought about, but, more important, the agencies could be a force in guiding the health providers, particularly hospitals, in reaching out to and providing neighborhoods and specific target populations with needed services. As the Macro Systems report says, "proponents usually argue for CON as a device for containing costs by allocating resources rationally and equitably. Facilities ... should be geographically distributed to meet community medical needs, and capital investments of dollars and manpower should reflect that distribution."[11]

As it developed, the health providers became the leaders and were heavily involved in the health-planning agencies responsible for implementing the CON and "1122" laws at the state and regional levels. They provided funds, staff time, experience, and guidance for the health planning agencies as much to avoid the threat of greater federal controls as to play a part in the cost containment and planning efforts that deeply affected them on a day-to-day basis. As one of the most heavily regulated industries in the United States, the hospital industry and its leaders were acutely aware that the regulatory trend could not be rolled back. The question was how they could best live with and control its impact on their activities.[12]

HOW HAVE THE CON/1122 LAWS WORKED?

The few major surveys and case studies of states with CON laws that have been reported thus far are inconclusive on the impact of CON or

"1122" laws on cost containment.[13] However, it is possible to identify some emerging trends that may offer clues about the future impact of these laws. The first part of this section will deal with case illustrations about CON laws and the second part, with the secondary effects of CON laws.

Bicknell reports on three years of experience with the Massachusetts CON program which began in 1972.[14] That law requires a CON for all new facilities with expenditures of $100,000 or more. Massachusetts at the time ranked seventeenth among states with 4.69 beds/1,000 persons and third in utilization of medical facilities at 2.81 days per person. There was recognition that alternatives to high cost medical facilities such as ambulatory care, higher occupancy rates, greater use of physician extenders, and changes in third party reimbursement policies would be required to reduce the use of hospitals. In the first three years there were 468 fewer beds approved for short term hospitals and approval of only 38% of the long term care bed requests. In contrast, there was very high approval rate of the 40 facility-improvement projects and the clinic proposals. Of the 15 appeals of the council's decisions, only one was reversed and that by the state agency itself upon its being remanded by the hearing body. On the surface, one could easily conclude that the CON program in Massachusetts was fairly successful in both containing costs and allocating services to areas of greatest need.

However, Bicknell was realistic in his assessment of the Massachusetts experience. First, he found that the cost overruns of the projects approved amounted to $112 million, which translates into higher per diem rates. Almost one-third of the projects had overruns of 26% or more over the original estimated costs. He further found that while denial of certificates prevents replacement or increase of beds, it does not remove excessive existing beds from service. Finally, the state agency failed to develop CON standards in order to make valid decisions. This meant that most decisions were based as much on rule of thumb or some generally accepted formula as they were on existing policy statements or the values of the persons voting on the individual projects. He concluded that "more than three years' experience ... tends to confirm that it (CON) is no panacea; alone, it is not equal to its broad assignment. When they can be identified, the diffuse factors bearing on the availability and costs of services fall beyond the scope of any one authority or agency within the State."[15]

In New Jersey, the Health Care Facilities Planning Act was passed in 1971 with the support of hospitals, Blue Cross, and consumer groups.[16] It became effective in August 1972. It gave broad powers to the state Department of Health to oversee the planning, construction, and licensing of new facilities, to set rates for third-party reimbursement by Blue Cross, and to monitor existing medical facilities to insure that they provide quality care in safe facilities. In 1971, compared to New York, Pennsylvania and the national average, New Jersey had a lower utilization rate and fewer beds per 1,000 population. This was attributed to the lack of a medical school and to the fact that residents went out of state (usually to New York City or Philadelphia) for secondary and tertiary levels of medical care. Still, Somers found that there were uneven levels of care, unnecessary care, and segments of the population with little or no care. Yet, through the "grandfathering" in of numerous projects before the effective date of the act, the slow process of writing the regulations, and the lack of adequate staff to perform the many tasks required for the law's implementation, Somers predicted that by 1977 there would be a surplus of 2,729 medical/surgical and 6,190 skilled nursing facility beds in New Jersey. She concluded, nonetheless, that it was too early to assess the law's effectiveness because of the extenuating circumstances under which the act was initially implemented. She felt that only one year's experience with CON was insufficient time to draw any serious conclusions.

In a recently published book on the CON process in New York, Rothenberg studied the changes in the state's bed capacity before and after the passage of Article 28 of the New York State Health Code in 1964.[17] She noted that "little could be attributed to the introduction of the CON legislation to regulating hospital bed expansion."[18] Her statistical analysis noted that the trend toward fewer, but larger hospitals was already well defined before the passage of Article 28 and that these trends merely continued after the passage of the law. For example, the number of hospitals with 50 or fewer beds decreased from 33 in 1960 to 18 in 1965. By 1970, after passage of the law, this decrease continued to 12 remaining fifty-bed hospitals. Rothenberg drew the inference that "facilities may have been located in places where their need was low," but offered no explanation for her finding.[19]

From these three studies, it appears that, as Bicknell suggests, CON legislation may not make a difference because there are too many other forces at work over which the CON laws have no influence. Yet, as Somers states, it may be too early to know what impact, if any, the CON laws will have on cost containment in the future. If one takes into account the five to seven years' lag between the pre-application period and the actual construction and opening of a hospital facility or major expansion, it may indeed be premature to evaluate the impact of CON laws on bed containment.

While it may be too early to offer more conclusive evidence of the CON or "1122" impact on cost containment, there are other secondary issues that stem from the regulatory process that may pose significant consequences for the health field. The four major issues which will be discussed briefly in this section are (1) that CON laws perpetuate the status quo, (2) that they tend to stifle competition and, by inference, innovation, (3) that the CON review boards and/or the committees are controlled by the medical providers much in the same way that regulators in other fields are frequently coopted by those they are supposed to be regulating, and (4) that in the competition between planning and regulation in the comprehensive health planning agencies, regulation receives more emphasis, staff, and status than do planning activities.

With respect to CON laws maintaining the status quo, all laws currently enacted are concerned with requiring a certificate for new facilities or services. They have grandfathered in and accepted the fact that existing services and facilities would not be affected by the CON laws. Thus, if a medical facility plan were completed for a region and the conclusion was that the area was overbedded for its population, that finding would effectively freeze the existing services until the situation altered. This would be the case whether the facilities were located to provide ready access to all segments of the population or not, or if some of the facilities were outmoded and required major renovation. If there were an oversupply of beds or services in the region, there would be a freeze on adding new services or facilities even if the needs of the population changed during the freeze.

Several writers have noted that the hospital associations have supported CON laws because the protection from new competitors who could be screened out through the CON process is worth the price they would have to pay for cost containment.[20] One writer notes that members of prepaid group plans (HMOs) use one-half to one-third less hospitalization than those who use physicians on a fee for service basis.[21] Yet, if the formulas used to determine bed needs are predicated on the proliferation of prepaid group plans, or HMOs, then the number of beds in the region would have to be reduced substantially or frozen for many years in the future at a major cost to hospitals in the region. However, committees reviewing CON requests are in a position to inhibit or prevent entry of threatening newcomers such as HMOs because they may run counter to the traditional methods of delivering medical services and may threaten to reduce the power of the private physician in his relationship to the hospital.

Havighurst, in particular, believes that the hospital facility and its administrators are used as straw men in the battle for cost containment. He believes the real battles involve the third-party financing mechanisms and the physicians who control the flow of patients to hospitals and determine, regardless of cost, what services will be used on behalf of their patients.[22] He notes that CON laws do not have any influence on either physician behavior or the rate setting mechanisms. Thus, while CON laws may well tend to stifle competition and inhibit innovation, cost stability may not be achieved if Havighurst and others are correct about the real sources of the problem.

In most states CON proposals are reviewed at both the regional and state levels. Whether the committee, as in the CHP "B" agencies, are mandated to have consumer majorities or not, it is the health providers who influence the course of the proceedings. Prior to the enactment of PL 93-641, health providers often contributed funds to the operation of these review bodies. Given their status, their powerful positions in the medical delivery system, and their potential for using the courts to overturn an unfavorable decision, the health providers either directly or indirectly are in a strong position to influence the outcome of CON decisions. The next chapter will show that the approval rate of the 36 geographic areas studied in a national survey was 90-95%. However this high approval rate came about, the implication is that health providers had to be playing an active role to be so successful.

With respect to the impact of regulatory activity on planning, there has been little question that the CHP "B" agencies were greatly understaffed because of inadequate funding by Congress. In 1972, almost all the "B" agencies were given the added responsibility of review and comment of both federally funded programs and projects requiring "1122" reviews. The supplementary funds provided by Congress to carry out this function were usually less than was needed to do a competent and complete review. To make up the difference, the "B" agencies tended further to delay development of their regional plans in order to meet the deadlines associated with review projects. Thus, staff was siphoned off from planning to regulatory functions.

However, the orientation of these two functions and the skills demanded of staff are so different that it is unlikely staff could easily move back and forth from one function to another. Planning is forward looking, review is reactive; planning is open-ended and dynamic, the regulatory process is rigid and formalistic with deadlines requiring definite decisions. Planning requires consensus building among those involved, whereas the review process is potentially adversary in nature.[23]

Furthermore, CHP "B" agencies tended to favor involvement in review of proposals to development of a regional plan. In the review process, decisions are made which lead to the eventual creation of real programs or to the construction or modernization of tangible medical facilities. It gives the agencies and their staffs a feeling of accomplishment, whereas planning seems nebulous and diffuse, and there is little hope of its culminating in real programs and services. It was thus not surprising that planning had a lower priority for staff and board. In many agencies, staff came to think of the regulatory process as planning for the community. Thus, staff, board, and health providers in CHP"B" agencies prefer to review CON proposals at the expense of planning.

In summary, it seems that CON and "1122" laws are still too new for their impact on cost containment to be determined. However, it does appear likely that the CON process is beginning to have serious secondary consequences such as maintaining the status quo in the health delivery system, stifling of competition and innovation, and substitution of regulation for planning as the primary activity of the regional planning agencies.

WHY CON'S IMPACT ON COST CONTAINMENT IS DOUBTFUL

As yet the real defect in the CON program has not been adequately addressed. Standards against which a facility or service can be evaluated are yet to be developed. There are two aspects to this problem. The first deals with the establishment of technical standards, which will be discussed in this section. The second, to be analyzed in the next section, concerns the normative factors involved in rendering decisions on projects. An often-heard planner's complaint is that no one pays attention to recommendations they make based upon objective standards they have developed. Instead, the planner too often finds that political influence is the standard that carries weight and is the one upon which decisions ultimately are made. Perhaps a look at these standards and criteria is required.

The most often utilized criterion for determining the need for a proposed facility or service has been the Hill-Burton methodology. This methodology is based upon population density and population projections and utilizes occupancy rates according to different service units. Medical/surgical, long-term, and pediatric/obstetrical are the units most commonly used by states in determining need. The calculations are then used to determine the number of beds needed to serve a region's population and are used as a standard for approving or denying requests for changes in medical facilities and services. Although the Hill-Burton formula has been criticized as simplistic and inaccurate, none of the other proposed methodologies has been more successful.[24] Instead, they all appear to have inherent limitations. Further, despite the use of sophisticated data and expertise, the outcomes appear no more accurate than those derived via Hill-Burton.

Although the virtue of the Hill-Burton formula is its simplicity, one should be aware of its limitations. The method assumes that the future will be the same as the present. Yet in a highly mobile population this assumption is not valid. One need only look at the New York City situation where, in 1976, 35 hospitals have been recommended for closure, a fact that would have been scoffed at five years earlier. Secondly, the Hill-Burton formula is so aggregative that it is unable to speak to needs for individual services within a medical facility. This is especially important because the great majority of requests for CON are for changes in service or modernization of existing facilities rather than for the establishment of new services or facilities. The formula is too broad in scope to offer much guidance to review committees. Third, the formula does not address the issue of whether or not the existing services are those which are needed at a given time. There may be too many beds in one part of the region and not enough physicians or outpatient facilities in another. The formula fails to consider the changing densities of population within a region, changes in population migration, or occurrences of medical problems that are unique to one part of a region. Finally, the formula does not identify if the services actually provided to the patient population are the appropriate ones. Studies in western New York indicated that among the elderly 75% were misplaced in mental institutions, 43% did not belong in the general hospitals where they were patients, and 24% were inappropriately placed in nursing homes.[25] However, in spite of these shortcomings, the Hill-Burton formula continues to be used because of its simple, easily employed methodology. As a broad framework, it works well. As a formula to meet changing needs, it leaves much to be desired.

If the Hill-Burton and other formulas fail to provide yardsticks for the need of proposed services, what about the CON laws themselves? Almost all experts agree that none of the laws contains scientifically based criteria or standards that offer the health providers or the review committees a tool for objective decisionmaking.[26] Criteria often used in the review of proposals usually include the following: (1) need of the population for the service, (2) the proposal's fiscal feasibility, (3) the availability of manpower to staff the service, (4) the competence and standing of the health provider, (5) the impact of the proposal on the rate structure and the environment, and so on. There are no standards that state whether or not a proposal is sound, needed, or fiscally viable. Millions of dollars are currently being spent by Professional Standard Review Organizations (PSROs) and consultants hired by the Bureau of Health Planning and

Resources Development, HEW, to develop appropriate standards for review. However, review committees cannot wait for the results of these efforts. They are required to make decisions on proposals presently confronting them. Whether there are objective standards or not, at least the CON laws have provided review committees with the necessary guidance and relevant questions. That is a starting point.

The health field has become prolific in its collection, analysis, evaluation, and use of data. The National Center for Health Statistics of HEW makes numerous surveys on the status of the health of the population, the utilization of medical services, the number, size, and location of medical facilities, and the number and type of medical manpower needed and used to provide services. One of the few functions on which the CHP"B" agencies scored well in HEW's assessment of their activities was the data function. The planning agencies in many cases were overwhelmed with the mountains of data that poured into them. However, their success in collecting the data was not matched by their use of it. It soon became apparent to the CHP"B" agencies and their review committees that good data were available, particularly general aggregated data, but that relevant data needed to shed light on specific proposals were either poor or nonexistent. Even when the review committees demanded these data from the sponsors of proposals, the usual response was that it was too time consuming and expensive to collect. How does one evaluate a proposal that calls for the addition of 25 mental health beds in a subarea of a region when the proposal does not have data to show how many people are waiting for service, what type of mental health services are needed, what type of alternative services are or could be provided, or whether there are enough psychiatrists or other mental health professionals to staff the new service?

The generalized data that are routinely collected do not usually shed light on questions such as these. The proposal's sponsor submits his best guestimates to satisfy the requirement, but that does not address the realities of the situation. The fact is that the health planners, the health providers, and the volunteer review committees do not know the facts. As Curran has noted, measurements of need usually require more relevant data than exist or have yet been collected.[27]

If the methods are not as useful as are needed, if the criteria and standards are too vague and general, and if the data are not available, then what is there to rely upon when making decisions on the CON requests? The answer is the use of comprehensive health plans for the regions. These contain goals and objectives. They specify the priorities the planning agencies agree are needed in the coming years. In addition, they identify the types of services, facilities, and locations necessary to implement the plan. With this type of detailed plan, the review committee has an important document against which to make decisions on CON/ "1122" proposals. Macro Systems' report points out the important relationship between planning and CON:

> Measurement and forecasting of need is indispensable to a CON program, as is a strategy which expresses a concept . . . of how providers should respond to that need. Both of these are planning functions, but without CON, planning of this type has been widely considered to be ineffective because planners have rarely had the means to enforce action which would carry out their plans.[28]

According to Macro Systems, the wedding between planning and regulation (CON reviews) is essential for both to be carried out effectively. Yet, the report goes on to note that the planning agencies are so overwhelmed with trying to keep up with their CON review responsibilities that they do not have the resources and time to undertake the vital task of developing these detailed, comprehensive plans. Almost no "B" agency and only a handful of states have developed satisfactory medical facility plans that could serve as a basis for objective decision-making.

Yet, millions of dollars worth of medical facility and service proposals are received each year and awarded CONs. Many of these services are vitally needed; many are not. One thing is certain—nature abhors empty spaces and so do medical providers. Parkinson's law states that hospital beds that are built tend to be used. That they are used does not mean that they are needed. Under circumstances where there is limited technical or scientific basis for making decisions on CON, just how are decisions made?

CON DECISIONMAKING IN THE ABSENCE OF PLANS OR STANDARDS

One of the techniques increasingly employed to forecast trends is the Delphi method. A series of experts, unknown to each other and in isolation, are asked to render their opinion on the future state of some specific issue. The responses are recorded and each participant receives the analysis of his colleagues and is further requested to respond to the analysis of these participants. After a series of these independent judgements, a consensus is eventually formed among the participants who remain anonymous to one another. In arriving at a consensus, it is obvious that experience, knowledge of the subject matter, and a capacity to be flexible in making tentative decisions are all involved in this method.

Using an adaptation of the Delphi method, review committees often make their decisions. Composed of consumers and providers, and supported by staff well acquainted with the proposal for a CON, the committee members bring to bear their individual and collective experience and knowledge of the proposal under review. They form initial judgements when they first receive and read the staff's summary of the proposal. They raise questions about the proposal, seek out answers, and directly confront both their own staff and the sponsor of the proposal with questions. They respond to each other. They reach out to community groups, both providers and consumers, who might be affected by the proposal. In this way, each person on the review committee over time renders his/her judgement on the proposal, and a consensus, often absent at the outset, forms until a vote and a decision can be made. The significant difference in the use of the Delphi method by the review committee is that the members know each other and are directly influenced by what each says and thinks. They often know the sponsor of the proposal. But, in the end a consensus is formed because the CON criteria guide their thinking, the available data assist the members to clarify opinions, and finally their own judgements of what is needed for the population affected by the proposal are brought to bear on the matter. The outcome of this process is a decision to approve or disapprove, amend, return with changes requested, or approve with conditions.

This process is referred to as a normative one in that the values of each member of the review committee, the planner, and the sponsor of the proposal are explicitly or implicitly involved in the final decision rendered. It is only when a compromise among different values can be found that a consensus forms. If one member sees the need for additional beds for a hospital wing, but another prefers that the funds be used to open an ambulatory care unit to serve a neighborhood with poor access to medical facilities, a compromise can sometimes be worked out. The hospital reduces its bed request to five and uses the funds for the other five beds to operate a mobile clinic several days a week in the neighborhood, to test the need for such a service. Whether the five additional beds are really needed or not may be a secondary issue to the review committee. It has used the hospital's request for more beds as a bargaining point to extend services to a neighborhood where its members believed a real need existed.

Rendering decisions based on normative values should not be viewed in a negative way. This method requires flexibility and the capacity to encompass differences of power and influence among groups as they each exert pressure to meet their own needs. Planning, too, is considered a normative process and is also supported by increasingly technical inputs (methods, data analyses, and reports). Cohen states that "the technical inputs into need assessment . . . are probably minor as compared to the subjective criteria that are invoked in determining whether a facility satisfies a local need."[29] He calls these the political realities but, at the same time, questions whether staff members engaged in the regulatory function are best suited to carry out the regulatory function so dependent upon precise decisions based on rigid formulas. Planners, on the other hand, work in an atmosphere where political bargaining occurs continuously. It is a role they are accustomed to performing. Consequently, it is the planner who is better equipped to handle the dynamics involved in rendering a CON decision. They have the skill and the flexibility necessary to make decisions in situations of uncertainty. It is for this reason that Cohen and others have urged planners to take a more active role in the review process.[30]

As already indicated, under the Partnership for Health Act, Congress did not award adequate funds for the health planning agencies to carry out their responsibilities without seeking supplementary assistance. In many cases, hospital associations and various medical organizations provided such assistance to these agencies. Quite often there was an unwritten understanding that the funds would be used to provide staff for regulatory reviews. In turn, the review committees had to take this fact into account when acting on a number of CON proposals. Under the new health planning act, PL 93-641, funds for planning and carrying out reviews continue to be inadequate. However, the new health systems agencies are prohibited from seeking supplementary funding from those directly involved in health services to avoid the conflict faced by the "B" agencies in the past. Thus, while this form of influence will be diminished, it is expected that it will be felt in other ways. One prominent student of the regulatory field predicts that if the CON laws fail, it will be because of the strong influence exerted by the hospital industry in health planning and on the CON process.[31]

There seems little question but that the health providers on the review committee tend to exert the greatest influence. In the past, health providers usually represented the majority of members on the state-wide councils that considered such decisions. This may be changing under the new health planning act where consumer majorities are mandated for both the regional and state health planning councils. This will probably not make a difference, because at the regional level consumers will be just as supportive as providers in approving any medical facilities or services requested for their areas. In the absence of a plan or other regional criteria, decisions are made on an ad hoc and project-by-project basis. It is considered sound planning as well as good politics when consumers representing a subarea of a region succeed in getting approval on a project for their community. It adds jobs and services to the community and is a source of personal status and influence to the consumer members or the committee. Under such circumstances, even if the consumers were not completely knowledgeable about all the ramifications of the proposal before them, they would tend to welcome the explanation and rationale offered by the project's sponsor and supported by other providers sitting on the review committee. The Macro Systems report on CON programs in 23 states led to the conclusion that in the absence of a plan, the judgements and status of providers on the review committee tended to overwhelm the consumer members.[32] The report states that "although provider groups generally are philosophically supportive, they understand instinctively that a highly sophisticated plan might well be inimical to their individual interests and intentions."[33]

What is obvious from these observations is that unless there is a major change of direction, it can be expected that the CON review process of the future will continue to be based on normative considerations. The health providers with the greatest stakes in the outcome of the process will continue to find ways, whether directly or indirectly, to perpetuate and maintain their influence. And past history indicates they will often find their most willing partners to be the consumer members of the review committees.

CON AND ITS LEGAL IMPLICATIONS

There are two types of legal threats that can evolve from the decisions rendered in the CON process. One is the process that permits the sponsor of a project and other specified parties (usually the regional planning agency or other parties subject to harm by the approval of the sponsor's project) to appeal a negative decision to a special hearing board or officer. The other is the appeal to the court system, which in some instances, carries with it a threat to the constitutionality of the CON law itself. In addition to the formal appeal mechanism, there is the sponsor's implied threat to take a negative decision through the judicial process.

As the CON process is regulatory, it is required to work in such a way that all parties seeking a decision from the various review committees be given an equal opportunity to receive favorable consideration on their proposals. If this due process is in any way arbitrary or open to questions of favoritism, the sponsor is in a position to appeal for a public hearing or a reconsideration of a negative decision. Where negative decisions are made without benefit of an approved health plan for the region or state, or where defined and known standards for determining need are not available, the sponsor is in a position to challenge the decisions by requesting a public hearing or taking the issue to the judiciary system. This is particularly true in cases of competing applicants. The Macro System report notes the danger to planners by suggesting that their credibility will be jeopardized when sophisticated and aggrieved parties appeal decisions by challenging the plan the decision was to implement, the criteria deriving from that plan, or the rationality of the administrative process applying those criteria.[34] If the sponsor felt that the review committee took too much or too little time in reviewing the application, that the information requested was too time consuming or expensive, yet was used as a basis for disapproval of the application, or that the review committee's interpretation of criteria or the identification of more efficient or effective alternative services changed from one applicant to the next, then the decision of the CON review committee was vulnerable and thus subject to challenge.

In Massachusetts, Bicknell noted that 15 appeals for public hearings were made over the first 19 months of the program.[35] Of these, only one was reversed and that by the CON agency itself when the case was remanded by the hearing agency for reconsideration. In all other cases, the applicant either lost his appeal or the appeal was withdrawn. Three of the 15 were filed for judicial review. The court upheld the planning agency's decision in two cases and dismissed the third for lack of sufficient evidence. The experience in Massachusetts seems to indicate that in spite of the potential threats of the overturning of unfavorable decisions, the appeal's hearing agency and the courts have usually upheld the CON agency. How typical the situation in Massachusetts may be is unknown, but it does raise questions about those who would give in to the threat of a sponsor to take an unfavorable decision to court by approving his CON rather than risk having the agency's negative decision overturned in court. If the reviewing agency feels threatened by a sponsor and responds in this passive manner, then the sponsor will have won a psychological victory. Yet the Massachusetts experience would indicate that the court's overruling of a sponsor's unfavorable decision is not likely. However, such threats on the part of sponsors can seriously interfere with the positive relationships that frequently develop between review committees and the various sponsors and thereby negatively affect the orderly CON process. Concern for the process as well as for the maintenance of positive relationships may mean more to the agency than any possible negative results from legal proceedings and lead to approval of questionable applications.

There have been several challenges to the constitutionality of the CON laws. Its constitutionality has been upheld in the states of New York, Kansas, and Oregon. In New York it was upheld on the grounds that it was necessary to "protect the public against too many hospitals and beds" that threatened the efficiency and effectiveness of the hospitals.[36] In Oregon, the challenge was to the agency's interpretation of its criteria by which it denied the applicant's request to relocate its hospital. The court upheld the CON agency's rights to interpret the criteria in the manner it did. In Kansas, the court overturned the decision of the CON reviewing agency on the ground that it was arbitrary in its discrimination against an applicant's request on the basis of its being a "for profit" hospital, whereas it had approved all of the not-for-profit applications.

The only state where the constitutionality of the CON law itself was struck down was in North Carolina where the North Carolina Supreme Court had ruled that the negative decision by the CON agency was an abridgement of the right of a business to compete for customers and its right to survive. It struck down the North Carolina law on the grounds that it created an unconstitutional monopoly on the part of the existing hospitals. In a special editorial, Elsasser of the American Hospital Association answered the arguments of the court by noting that (1) the hospital industry is not like other industries because the patient is not free to go to any hospital of his/her choice, but rather is directed to a hospital at the discretion of his/her doctor, and (2) contrary to the thinking of the court, which stated that any business venture should permit a firm to compete and go bankrupt if it fails, Elsasser noted that the pricing structure of health care protected medical facilities from bankruptcies by having the third party payor make up the difference to underutilized hospitals by raising the per diem rate to insure that the hospital has sufficient income to balance its budget. Unlike other businesses, inefficiency is rewarded in the health care field.[37] This is based on the humanistic principle that medical care is considered a public trust in which the health care and safety of the patient is placed above profits.

Although the North Carolina decision came as a shock to states with CON legislation, the review of the decision and the prior favorable court decisions in other states permitted hospital legal experts to view the North Carolina decision as idiosyncratic and questioned its role in determining the future direction of CON laws. Nonetheless, the ambiguity of many of the states' criteria, the delegation of authority in some instances to private planning agencies, and the possibility of the CON agency's using manipulation and disapproval to foster certain outcomes such as the closing of a hospital or the negotiating of a desired merger are issues that may continue to subject CON laws to future constitutional challenges.

The American Hospital Association, which generally supports CON laws, cautions its member hospitals to "proceed with extreme caution when contemplating the support of a court challenge of your state's CON law. If it does not suit your needs or if the process is weak or unwieldy, think seriously about supporting legislation to amend the statute."[38] The AHA fears that a court challenge may unwittingly lead to a state's CON law's being declared unconstitutional, as occurred in North Carolina.

RECOMMENDED ALTERNATIVES FOR COST CONTAINMENT AND MEETING THE HEALTH NEEDS OF THE REGION

Up to this point, the discussion has raised a number of questions about the effectiveness of CON laws to contain the rapidly escalating costs of medical care. The picture is unclear because most states that have passed such laws have done so too recently to permit an evaluation of their impact. It takes many years for the true impact of a program to be felt. Yet, the many students of CON laws are frankly skeptical about its ultimate outcome and have suggested alternative methods for dealing with the problem of cost containment. In this section a brief review of these alternative recommendations will be presented.

There are two main focuses that require attention in examining these alternatives:

1. What effect are they likely to have on cost containment?
2. How will they meet the population's need for medical care?

Self-Regulation

This was the primary position of the hospital industry prior to the CON laws of 1964. With the assistance of the federal government, area-wide health facility councils (mainly controlled by hospital officials and trustees) were created to develop facility plans for which voluntary compliance with their goals and objectives was required. The aim was to coordinate services and allocate them in a more rational manner. This method has obviously not worked for the several reasons noted in earlier sections of this chapter. With the trend toward increasing regulation by the state and federal governments, it is unlikely that the industry will find itself deregulated and given a second chance. The positive effect of this strategy has been to produce a high quality of medical care for that large portion of the population who could afford its services. Unfortunately, there were many other segments who could not afford these services and accordingly did not benefit. Neither did this strategy do anything to reduce the rapid escalation of medical costs.

Self-Regulation with Some Federal Guidelines

This strategy recognizes the problems of the medical system's failure to use scarce resources most efficiently and to provide basic services to all segments of the population. It was recognized that for the medical care system to be more responsive to economic incentives, there would have to be much prodding from the federal government. Advocates of this approach have favored such strategies as the establishment of health care corporations or HMOs, federal payment of care for low income groups, the use of some form of prospective budgeting to limit institutional costs, and the sharing of expensive specialized services with other institutions. These strategies would tend to foster high quality care at lowest costs. The problem has been for the federal government to define the incentives required to induce the existing medical care system to accept this type of restructuring. Thus far, the basic medical system continues to prevail in spite of the increasing constraints and regulations placed on it. Without some form of national health insurance and federal mandate requiring a change in the organization of the medical system, this approach is unlikely to change direction. The system has already shown itself to be adaptive to external pressures without basically altering itself.

Franchising

This strategy would give to the state the public regulation of hospitals based on a plan devised by the medical care system. The state regulatory body would then grant a license to a hospital to carry out part of the assigned functions identified in the plan and provide the requisite services to all persons within the assigned geographic area. This would assure that all residents had access to quality service. The system would be designed to foster services at the lowest cost possible. The threat of losing the franchise would be incentive enough for the medical providers to economize wherever possible. This strategy is similar to the one above, except that it has state instead of federal guidance and it retains the traditional delivery system instead of restructuring it. It would be a form of voluntary operation of a medical institution within a limited state-planned framework and general guidelines. Such a system would probably result in the provision of services to all persons within a prescribed community. However, it is doubtful if the medical institutions would have incentives to economize when it is guaranteed a patient population and becomes a sanctioned medical monopoly in the provision of service in its geographic area. Without a change in the ways physicians practice, are paid for their services, and control the entry of patients into the medical system, the medical facility would be helpless to institute changes without an external mandate from the state or federal government. Costs of medical care would likely rise even faster under this plan.

State-Federal Control of Hospital Care

In this strategy, there would be no halfway measure of voluntary activity on the part of the medical system. The state and/or federal governments would impose strict controls on the medical system through a series of regulations that would, in effect, make them wards of the government. They would be treated as a typical public utility and be accountable to the government in lowering costs and providing treatment to all persons on an equal basis. The government would have to guarantee payment of all patient costs so that some form of national health insurance would be required. Because the medical system would still be operated by the private sector, it would have to provide either an incentive to the hospital administrators and its medical staff to comply voluntarily or to install a large scale monitoring system to insure compliance with governmental standards. Under this system, there may be a lowering of quality of service in order to live within the price structure set by the government, or there may be high quality service at very high costs to the taxpayer. It is unlikely both goals could be reached simultaneously under this system as there are no real incentives for the administrators or physicians to strive for cost containment and still permit them to render quality care for all in need of it.

Quasi-Regulation and Planning in a Government/Private Sector Partnership

This essentially is the strategy of PL 93-641, the National Health Planning and Resources Development Act of 1974. This strategy requires a comprehensive plan for the region and state to be developed before federal funds would be allocated to provide medical services and facilities. A mandatory federal CON program would be developed in every state with minimum federal criteria and procedures. Need would be initially determined by the CON application's fit to the priority ranking of the health system's goals and objectives. In time, standards will be developed to determine need for different services, the quality of the service provided, and the utilization of and access to the services. In this way, a technical-planning-legal framework would be developed to guide the medical care system. The planning and health care systems would still be largely in the control of the not-for-profit medical institutions. There would be no controls placed on the physician, no changes in the traditional physician-patient relationship nor in the manner of physician payments. This system would probably be both more efficient and more effective in serving the patient population. However, it is doubtful whether this will result in any great reduction in medical costs as there is no incentive for the physician to alter his way of working with patients or his use of medical facilities and services. Likewise, unless the hospitals were guaranteed payment for all the patients they served, there is no incentive for them to serve those too poor to pay for services and not eligible for government-sponsored medical insurance. Without some form of national health insurance and a restructuring of incentives as prepaid group medical care, there would not likely be any basic change in the medical delivery system or the patient population it serves.

As can be seen from these alternative solutions, the CON laws represent only one among a number of approaches to reducing or containing costs of medical care and at the same time fostering a more equitable distribution of services. It is for this reason that CON as a regulatory function will probably be linked, as in PL 93-641, to a regional health plan. It is the health plan and its statement of priorities that provide the mandate to render services to the people of the region. The plan can be used as a legal tool to force compliance on the part of the medical providers to promote those services called for in the plan. In this way, CON becomes a positive regulatory tool guided by a plan to promote both cost containment and improved allocation of resources. Whether these twin goals will be achieved under the regulatory-planning strategy is questionable.

As an introductory chapter, this has been an attempt to provide an overview of the major issues impacting on CON laws. Chapter two is an examination of the latest findings of how the CON laws have worked in the United States. Chapter three discusses the CON and "1122" sections of PL 93-641. It tells the health providers what is expected of them and what the law means. Chapter four provides a legal interpretation of CON under PL 93-641 along with a detailed discussion of some of the constitutional issues involved in the act. It will identify areas the provider should be aware of. Chapter five identifies the latest methods for determining community needs and their relationship to the Health Systems Plan and the Annual Implementation Plan which the new Health Systems Agencies must produce. Under the new law, institutional planning and implementation must go hand in hand with regional health planning. This chapter will assist the health provider in understanding that relationship. Chapter six discusses public accountability as it relates to the regulatory function. It also deals with how the normative aspects of planning influence and are influenced by the regulatory factors with which health providers must cope. The final chapter assesses the current status of CON and what must be done to make the regulatory process a more dynamic and relevant tool for encouraging cost containment while providing needed services.

Notes

3. Anne Somers, *Hospital Regulation: The Dilemma of Public Policy* (Princeton: Princeton University, Industrial Relations Section, 1969).

4. Clark C. Havighurst, ed., *Regulating Health Facilities Construction* (Washington, D.C.: American Enterprise Institute for Public Policy Research, 1974).

5. David F. Drake, "Public Utility: Its Meaning for Hospitals," *Trustee* 26, no. 4 (April 1973): 1-9.

6. Ibid., p. 6.

7. Richard T. Fox, "Are Controls a Necessary Evil?" *Hospital Progress* 55 (August 1974): 6.

8. Ibid., p. 12.

9. Roger N. Whiting, "Suggested Organizational Changes for the Hospital Industry," *Health Services Reports* 88, no. 8 (October 1973): 743-749.

10. Ibid., p. 749.

11. Macro Systems, Inc., *The Certificate of Need Experience: An Early Assessment,* (Silver Spring, Maryland: Vol I: Summary Report, April 1974), p. 8.

12. See Clark C. Havinghurst, "Regulations in the Health Care System" *Hospitals* 48 (June 16, 1974): 65-70 for a provocative treatment of this subject.

13. See William J. Bicknell and Diana C. Walsh, "The Certificate of Need: The Massachusetts Experience," *The New England Journal of Medicine,* May 15, 1975, pp. 1054-1061; Eleanore Rothenberg, *Regulation & Expansion of Health Facilities: The C/N Experience in New York State* (New York: Praeger, 1976): Anne Somers, *State Regulations of Hospitals and Health Care: The New Jersey Story* (Chicago: Blue Cross Reports, No. 11 Research Series, July 1973); Macro Systems, Inc., op. cit; William J. Curran, Richard J. Steele and Ellen W. Ober, "Government Intervention on Increase," *Hospitals* 49 (May 16, 1975): 57-61; and Patrick O'Donoghue, *Evidence About the Effects of Health Care Regulation* (Denver, Colorado: Spectrum Research Inc., 1974), Chap. IV. These studies represent only some of the recently published reports on evaluations of certificate of need laws.

14. Bicknell and Walsh, op. cit.

15. Ibid., p. 1060.

16. See Somers, op. cit.

17. Rothenberg, op. cit.

18. Ibid., p. 3 of Rothenberg summary of published work, mimeo.

19. Ibid., p. 20 of summary.

20. See Macro Systems, Inc., op. cit., p. 9; Havighurst, op. cit., p. 66; and Eddie Correira, "Public Certificate of Need for Health Facilities," *AJPH* 65, no. 3 (March 1975): 264.

21. Correira, op. cit., p. 262.

22. Havighurst, op. cit., p. 67.

23. See Macro Systems, Inc., op. cit., for a more detailed discussion of the relationship between planning and review functions.

24. See P.F. Gross, "Urban Health Disorders, Spatial Analysis and the Economics of Health Facility Location," *International Journal of Health Services* 2, no. 1 (1972): 63-84 for a concise and excellent analysis of seven different methods.

25. Ibid., pp. 72-73.

26. See Curran, et al., op. cit., and Macro Systems, Inc., op. cit., for the best discussion of this issue.

27. Curran, et al., op. cit.

28. Macro Systems, Inc. op. cit., p. 14.

29. Harris S. Cohen, "Regulating Health Care Facilities: The Certificate of Need Process Re-Examined," *Inquiry* X (September 1973): 8.

30. See Correira, op. cit. and Macro Systems, Inc., op. cit. as examples of experts taking this position.

31. Havighurst, op. cit., p. 68.

32. Macro Systems, Inc., op. cit., pp. 29-30.

33. Ibid., p. 28.

34. Ibid., p. 31.

35. Bicknell and Walsh, op. cit., pp. 1057-58.

36. Curran et al., op. cit., p. 174 for a discussion of these cases.

37. Peter J. Elsasser, "Questions/ Answers: C/ N No Longer Useful?" *Hospitals* 48 (July 1, 1974): 26.

38. Ibid., p. 26.

Chapter 2

The Efficiency and Effectiveness of Health Care Capital Expenditures and Service Controls: An Interim Assessment[1]

Carolyn Harmon

INTRODUCTION

One of the most striking aspects of health care capital expenditure and services controls is the rapidity with which they have become accepted as state and federal policy. Prior to 1970, only five state certificate of need laws had been enacted and no such mandatory controls existed in federal law; four years later a total of 24 states had enacted CON statutes and the federal government had adopted a state-option form of control in Sec. 1122 of the Social Security Act. Thirty-seven states entered into contracts with the federal government to implement the Sec. 1122 program, with the result that only three states in the U.S.—Texas, Vermont, and West Virginia—had no form of health care capital expenditure and services controls by mid-1974. With the enactment of PL 93-641 in January of 1975, CON programs became mandatory for all states.

Given the number of variables thought to affect health care costs—e.g., patterns of utilization, unionization of health care personnel, types of costs covered by third-party reimbursement systems, and state rate control, to name but a few—assessment of the relative contribution of CON controls to overall health care cost control presents formidable methodological problems, and no definitive answer to this question is likely in the near future.

What can and should be assessed at this early stage of development of health care capital expenditure and services controls are:

1. the objectives, coverage, resources, and organization of state regulatory systems—i.e., the capacity of states to prevent creation of unneeded facilities and services;

2. the actual effect of regulatory decisions on the health care system, with respect to both the number and cost of unneeded projects denied and changes in the balance of high and low cost services in the area;

3. the efficiency and fairness of state regulatory procedures;

4. the hidden costs of such controls.

The purpose of this chapter is to report on the status of both CON and Sec. 1122 controls with respect to each of these issues as determined by a study of 20 sample states by Lewin & Associates, Inc., which was conducted from September 1974 to September 1975. These data suggest the nature of the base on which PL 93-641 must build and the areas of weakness to which the federal government must direct its attention if state CON laws are to achieve the objectives of this legislation.

STUDY DESIGN

The study involved a field survey of a sample of 20 states and 35 area-wide (314b) health planning agencies within these states. In selecting the sample, states were grouped by type of control (CON only, 1122 only, CON and 1122, and no controls other than voluntary review).

States were then selected in rough proportion to the total number of states with each type of control(s), taking geographic distribution into account. To the extent feasible, one urban and one rural area-wide health planning agency was sampled within each state. States included in the study are shown in Table 2-1.[2]

Data were obtained in each state through interviews with state and local review agencies, other state officials, third party payers, and provider groups and through review of agency files. Data included:

- *Individual project* type, cost, sponsor, length of time for review, and agency decisions
- *Review processes*, including number of levels of review, participants in review decisions, type of analyses performed, timing, and provisions for due process
- *Review tools*, including health care plans, data, and review criteria
- *Agency resources*, including budget and staffing characteristics
- *Participant views*, including the purpose and perceived effects of CON or 1122, the adequacy of health care supply, and attitudes toward certain classes of providers

In addition, the provisions of CON laws in the sample and all other states were identified through review of prior studies.[3,4]

TABLE 2-1
STUDY SAMPLE
(Sample States Are Italicized)

PRIOR CES CONTROLS	1122 ADOPTED		1122 NOT ADOPTED
CON	Colorado	New York	Arizona
	Florida	North Dakota	*California*
	Kentucky	Oklahoma	Connecticut
	Maryland	*Oregon*	District of Columbia
	Michigan	South Carolina	*Kansas*
	Minnesota	*Virginia*	Massachusetts
	Nevada	Washington	Rhode Island
	New Jersey		South Dakota
			Tennessee
Voluntary Planning Only	Alabama	*Missouri*	*Illinois*
	Alaska	*Montana*	*Texas*
	Arkansas	Nebraska	*West Virginia*
	Delaware	New Hampshire	Vermont
	Georgia	New Mexico	
	Hawaii	North Carolina	
	Idaho	*Ohio*	
	Indiana	*Pennsylvania*	
	Iowa	Wisconsin	
	Louisiana	Utah	
	Maine	Wyoming	
	Mississippi		

These data, while not statistically representative of CON and 1122 systems, provide the most comprehensive assessment of the implementation of health care capital expenditure and services controls to date. What they suggest with respect to each of the four major issues identified above is reported in the following sections.

OBJECTIVES AND CHARACTERISTICS OF CON AND 1122 SYSTEMS

One goal of the Lewin research was to identify and measure the principal goals and salient characteristics of state CON and Section 1122 programs as a way of determining the capacity of state and area agencies to prevent the creation of unnecessary health facilities and services. In particular, the study focused on measuring the following objectives and characteristics of state and area review programs:

- The extent to which state and areawide CON and 1122 agencies share the federal cost control objective

- Coverage and sanctions of state CON laws as compared to Sec. 1122
- The organization of the review process
- Review criteria and data used by review agencies

The results of this aspect of the study are discussed below.

CON and Section 1122 Agency Objectives

In forming conclusions about the capacity of CON and 1122 agencies to prevent unnecessary capital expenditures and services, it was necessary first to determine what these agencies were trying to achieve.

TABLE 2-2
COMPARISON OF COVERAGE AND THRESHOLDS FOR SECTION 1122 AND STATE CON PROGRAMS

COVERAGE	Sec. 1122	No. of State CON Laws that Meet or Exceed 1122
1. Providers		
a. Hospitals	X	23
b. Nursing Homes	X	23
c. Ambulatory Care	X	19
2. Expenditures for Plant		
a. Acquisition	X	N/A
b. New Construction	X	24
c. Expansion	X	21
d. Renovation	X	21
e. Replacement	X	18
3. Expenditures for Equipment		
a. New Purchase	X	17
b. Replacement	X	13
4. Bed Change		
a. Additions	if capital expenditure	24
b. Reductions	if capital expenditure	13
5. Service Change		
a. New	if capital expenditure	18
b. Expansion	if capital expenditure	11
c. Reduction	if capital expenditure	6
d. Cessation	if capital expenditure	8
THRESHOLD	$100,000 or any amount if capacity/ service change	16*

* Includes all states that express thresholds as % of operating costs

The primary objective of the federal government in supporting CON regulation is to contain health costs by preventing the development of unnecessary health facilities and services. However, the findings from the 20 sample states suggest that fewer than half of the state and area agencies that administered Sec. 1122 and CON controls shared the federal commitment to cost containment.

In some states, this could be explained by the existence of formal rate regulation, which is looked to as the primary tool for containing health costs. In the main, however, discussions with these agencies suggested that their commitment to cost containment was diluted by two factors. (1) The link between CON or 1122 controls and cost containment, while accepted, was poorly understood. Moreover, most agencies did not have data about total health care costs for their state or area and, therefore, could not measure or project the impact of review decisions on these costs. (2) Improving the quality and distribution of health services and facilities were more pressing local issues than the total cost of health services and the impact of these costs on public and consumer budgets.

Other objectives for controls that were defined by states and area agencies in addition to or in lieu of cost containment were usually the secondary federal policy goals of increased public participation and improved provider planning. As might be expected, there was a somewhat greater commitment to public participation at the area level. In addition, most state agencies viewed CON or 1122 controls as a means of promoting the development of health resources in underserved areas, and three states specified that such controls were intended to insure the financial viability of existing providers. It must be concluded that state capacity for preventing unnecessary facilities and services, as measured by the agencies' own objectives and comprehension of the cost implications of their decisions, is a matter for serious federal concern.

Scope of Coverage, Thresholds, and Sanctions of CON and 1122

The "coverage" of Sec. 1122 and state CON laws refers to the types of providers and the types of facility and service changes that are regulated. "Threshold" refers to the size of the capital expenditure or service change required to trigger the review process. Table 2-2 summarizes Sec. 1122 coverage and thresholds and compares them to the provisions of the 24 state CON laws in operation as of June 1974.

Section 1122 covers all major classes of health care institutions, any capital expenditure that exceeds $100,000, or any capital expenditure of any amount that increases or decreases capacity or service. This coverage is more comprehensive than many state CON laws with respect to replacement of equipment and reduction in beds or services. However, the majority of state CON laws appeared to provide adequate authority for prevention of unnecessary beds and services if Sec. 1122 is viewed as a standard. (Only a few states which had CON laws prior to 1122 adopted the latter program to improve their coverage. The remainder adopted 1122 primarily to obtain federal funding for regulatory program administration.) In addition, 13 state CON laws had more stringent thresholds than Sec. 1122 in that they regulated capacity and service changes whether or not a capital expenditure was involved.

The most obvious and apparently significant difference between Sec. 1122 and state CON laws is the type of sanction applied to enforce review decisions. Under Sec. 1122, capital costs (principal, interest, depreciation, etc.) incurred without state approval would not be reimbursed by the Medicare, Medicaid, and Maternal and Child health programs. State CON rulings, on the other hand, are enforced through denial of an operating license, court injunctions, and fines. However, it was found that providers typically complied with negative review decisions regardless of the type of sanction available to the state. Thus, the majority of states can be said to have had adequate legal authority to prevent unnecessary capital expenditures and services prior to enactment of PL 93-641.

The Organization of the Review Process

A basic assumption underlying CON controls is that decisions about capital expenditures and service changes in the health industry should not be the exclusive province of the providers of health care. Instead, because of the effect of these decisions on the public welfare, these controls have been established to bring decisions about health care resources into a more public, community-oriented setting. In addition, such controls are looked to as a way of requiring economic analysis of health resource allocation decisions which, because factors such as third party reimbursement and publicly subsidized capital financing distort economic incentives in the health industry, are not subject to the usual rigors of the market place.

It is important, therefore, to know how CON and 1122 reviews have been conducted and the extent to which different ways of organizing the review process enhance public participation and insure opportunity for careful analysis of proposals. The process followed in conducting CON and 1122 reviews can be characterized as having two basic phases: (1) a pre-review phase during which proposals are defined and applications prepared and filed and (2) the formal review and decision process, which typically takes place at both the area and state levels. Characteristic types of organization and procedures within each phase are described below.

Application and Completeness Reviews

Three of the nine sample CON states—Michigan, New Jersey, and New York—did not make formal rulings on or give notice that an application was complete and accepted for review. As will be seen in the discussion of efficiency and due process, this appears to have implications both for the duration of reviews and for due process.

Although the form and content of the CES review applications being used by the sample states varied enormously, most were poorly designed from the point of view of both the applicant and the agency. The major problems observed include the following:

- *Poor design and organization.* In some states, it was necessary to read almost the entire application to determine the exact nature of the proposal and sponsor.
- *Ambiguous information requests.* A surprising number of applications ask for narrative responses to questions such as, "How does this proposal meet community health needs?"
- *Failure to require, in verifiable form, crucial financial and operating data.* Applications sometimes do not clearly require such basic data as current and prior utilization, proposed financing costs and current debt load, effects on rates, proposed staffing, etc. Financial data in particular were deficient (e.g., major hospital expansions were reviewed without obtaining even an uncertified financial statement).

As evidence of the deficiencies in CON and 1122 applications, it was impossible to determine the dollar value for nearly a third of the nearly 3,000 project files examined. Some of these were pending while further information was obtained from the provider, and others may not have involved a dollar outlay (e.g., closing beds with no expense requires approval in some states); however, a majority of the proposals without cost data clearly did involve some expenditure.

Formal Review and Decision Process

Staff and committee reviews. Two basic approaches were used by area agencies: in one, joint staff-council member task forces were assigned to review each proposal or all proposals of a certain type (e.g., hospitals) and recommend action to the facilities committee or full council; in the other, agency staffs conducted the analysis and presented materials for committee and council review. We found no clear basis for selecting one over the other except local preference.

An issue of great concern in a few agencies was whether staff should make recommendations or merely present data and analysis. While there was evidence that where staff did make recommendations the staff process was superior, there is again no clear basis other than local preference for choosing between the two approaches.

Levels of review. At the area and sometimes the state level, proposals passed through several levels of committees before final action was taken. For example, there might be subarea committees as well as the area-wide council in each county and major municipality. If there were project review subcommittees at both levels, there would have been four levels of review by the time the final area agency decision was made. Ordinarily, all involved public meetings and all but the area-wide council session were likely to entail a more or less formal presentation by the sponsor of the proposal. The result was that, by the time final state action was taken, there might have been five or six separate levels of committee review.

Most CON statutes establish a state level council to review and recommend action on proposals. However, among 1122-only states, where the use of councils is optional, relatively few states consulted with councils on individual projects and several of those that started out with councils had since ended council participation as being unworkable due to time demands.

Public participation in the review process. The meaning of public, or consumer, participation in health planning and review has long been a subject of dispute and/or confusion. At one level, consumer membership on review boards is seen as "public participation," and whether the consumers are to be elite (middle-class, usually professional) or "representative of the community" (a euphemism for poor and social/ethnic minorities) has been a source of conflict in the years since 1965. If the area agencies we visited are representative, this conflict has, for the most part, been resolved in favor of the elite consumer.

Most CON states and all Sec. 1122 states required consumer majorities on decisionmaking bodies involved in the review process. However, having a consumer majority or agency councils does not, by itself, insure effective consumer participation in review decisions. Therefore, to measure consumer and provider participation in CON and 1122 decisions, we examined board attendance reports for the sample agencies. We were able to obtain these data in six of the states that used councils and 23 of 36 area agencies. The purpose of this examination was to determine how often providers were in the majority at meetings in which final action was taken on proposals. We found that providers were in the minority in 47% of all area council decision-making meetings and in 26% of such meetings at the state level. More striking is the fact that more than half of the 23 area agencies had provider majorities at more than 50% of their meetings.

Equally disturbing, a number of agencies actually permitted or encouraged provider-dominated primary review committees to insure "expertise." Other agencies claimed that, regardless of the proportion of providers present at decision meetings, consumers would typically follow the lead of providers whom they perceived as having more competence. (This perception was frequently justified, as few agencies had systematic orientation processes for consumer council members.) Actual provider vs. consumer voting patterns did not appear to occur in any agency. Thus, the problem of insuring a meaningful direct role for consumers in health care capital expenditure and service decisions was still unresolved at the time of the study.

With respect to more general public participation in and awareness of the CON or 1122 process, most CON states and all Sec. 1122 states were required to give public notice that a proposal was under review so that interested members of the community could communicate with the review agency. Most, but not all, agencies honored this requirement through routine paid public notices in local or statewide newspapers. Agencies had done little to educate the media to the CON or 1122 process or to the cost implications of their decisions so that, with few exceptions, media coverage tended to be spotty and uninformed.

Most, but not all, area level agencies held public hearings on proposals, but reported that such meetings were poorly attended except in highly controversial and emotion-laden cases (e.g., proposed closing of a hospital maternity ward). While most of the agencies surveyed accepted public participation as a good principle, they were for the most part, at a loss as to how to bring about such participation. It would seem that, if the agencies themselves better understood the relationship between health care capital expenditures and costs to the consumer, they would be better able to generate the public participation and support needed to insure the successful implementation of PL 93-641.

Area-state roles and relationships. California and Kansas assigned final decisionmaking authority, short of appeal, to the area agencies. Except for these two states, de jure area-state relations were much the same in all states regardless of the type of controls in place. However, de facto area-state relationships varied among the states quite substantially, principally in terms of which level dominates the substantive analysis and decisionmaking process. In general, states with long established

CON programs were more likely to conduct independent analyses of provider proposals and were less reliant on area-wide agency analyses and recommendations.

It could be concluded, on the basis of these data, that states with both CON and 1122 controls typically have provided adequate formal opportunities for analysis of proposals by a variety of groups, although the process generally has failed to include the broader public or insure meaningful consumer majorities in the review process. Deficiencies in the information base contained in project applications, moreover, set serious limits on the capacity of reviewers to perform effective analyses or make reasoned review decisions. This factor, along with the deficiencies in agency data, plans, and criteria discussed below suggests that implementation of PL 93-641 should focus on the content more than on structure of the review process.

Review Criteria and Data Resources

The capacity of an agency to make an informed decision on a health care facility or service proposal and, in doing so, to assure that it knows and can inform the community about the impact of its decisions, is heavily dependent on the review criteria and data resources of the agency. Thus, it is extremely significant and disturbing that few review agencies at either the state or area levels had adequate need projections, review criteria, or data resources with which to conduct the review function. Most state and area agencies relied on Hill-Burton need projections which were based on obsolete data and which, in the opinion of the agencies themselves, were inappropriate for reviews. Criteria for review of special services were rare (Table 2-3) except for X-ray equipment and renal dialysis services. The need projections and criteria that did exist generally reflected a "no change" assumption about the present configuration of the health delivery system, although there was little evidence that alternative configurations had been considered. Moreover, there was a widespread tendency to apply criteria in reviews that were not made explicit, e.g., preferences for "full service hospitals" or opposition to proprietary providers.

The lack of complete and reliable data was even more commonplace among review agencies than the absence of review criteria. For example, of all the data elements required for health planning and regulation, acute care bed supply data is the most easily obtained. Yet, nearly half of the sample state agencies relied on hospital bed data that were at least two years old. The situation with respect to long term care (LTC) beds, specialty services, and equipment was much worse. Current, reliable utilization data were practically nonexistent.

TABLE 2-3
DISTRIBUTION OF STANDARDS DEVELOPED BY STATE AND AREA AGENCIES

SPECIALTY SERVICES AND EQUIPMENT	STATE	AREAS
Hospital Specialty Beds	4	7
Psychiatric Beds	2	3
Scanners Supervoltage	4	11
Renal Dialysis	7	12
ICU/CCU	4	5
Home Health Care	2	4
SurgiCenter	—	2
Other Outpatient	3	8
Rehabilitation Services	4	5
Cardiac Surgery/Cath.	4	9
X-Ray Equipment	2	4
Other Equipment Services	4	4
Number in Cell	20	36

Except in one or two states which have state-administered rate controls, data about health costs, prices, and expenditures were simply not available. Similarly, few agencies possessed data on which to base an analysis of the proposed cost of developing new facilities and equipment.

In a few instances, the lack of adequate review criteria is a function of the state-of-the art in health planning. For example, there appears to be no fully developed or widely accepted methodology for projecting the effects on acute inpatient facilities and services of expanding the supply of ambulatory care and long term care facilities. Moreover, there is a continuing need for the development of review criteria in response to new technology (e.g., the EMI and "whole body" scanners).

However, since nearly all types of need projections and criteria required for effective regulation had been developed by at least some agencies—and a few agencies had most of what they needed—it is clear that in most cases the obstacles to developing criteria and data resources are not technological. Instead, the problem is more often a lack of management leadership and competence and/or inadequate resources. In addition, few agencies had the authority to require providers to make regular reports of the data needed for effective health planning and regulation.

While PL 93-641 promises to improve agency access to current provider data, these findings suggest that there is an overwhelming lack of capacity to plan for change or to understand and make use of data among existing review agencies.

THE OUTCOMES AND EFFECTIVENESS OF CES CONTROLS

This section summarizes the principal findings and conclusions concerning the outcomes and effectiveness of CON and 1122 reviews based on an analysis of:

- The characteristics, disposition, and implications for the health care system of nearly 3,000 proposals reviewed by the sample states and areas
- The performance of the sample states and areas in deterring unnecessary capital investment
- The factors associated with success in this regard

Nature of Proposals and Decisions

During the survey period, the 17 sample states that had formal controls in operation received or acted on a total of 2,891 proposals. The number and average cost of these proposals by type of institution and type of expenditure proposed is reported in Table 2-4.[5] An analysis of the characteristics and disposition of these proposals, and discussions with agencies and providers, indicated that regardless of the type of controls in place, states approved more than 93% of all projects submitted and 90% of the dollar expenditures proposed.

New facilities represented a small proportion of the hospital proposals received by all states and had a comparatively low approval rate; expansion proposals were a large proportion of all hospital proposals and had a comparatively high approval rate. Overall, hospital proposals of all kinds were approved somewhat more often (90.5% of 1,134 proposals reviewed) than those sponsored by nursing homes (85.2% of 842 proposals) or other types of health care institutions (90.1% of 202 proposals). These data support the impression gained through the survey that, although providers and regulators were in general agreement that new hospitals are seldom needed, there was little opposition to expanding existing institutions. While less costly than new facilities in the short run, the expansion of existing institutions revealed a steady and substantial increase in hospital capacity, which would tend to exacerbate the maldistribution of health care resources.

The fact that nursing home proposals were denied more frequently than those for hospitals and other facilities—free-standing clinics, psychiatric care facilities, etc.—may be due to several factors. Competitive nursing home proposals, i.e., two or more similar proposals where only one is likely to be approved, were common, whereas direct competition

TABLE 2-4
DISTRIBUTION OF PROPOSED EXPENDITURES BY TYPE OF CHANGE PROPOSED—ALL SUBMISSIONS

	TOTAL PROJECTS			MODERNIZATION		MODERNIZATION/EXPANSION		EXPANSION		NEW FACILITY		EQUIPMENT		OTHER	
	No.	Total $(000)	Avg. $(000)	No. (%)	Avg. $(000)	No. (%)	Avg. $(000)	No. (%)	Avg. $(000)	No. (%)	Avg. $(000)	No. (%)	Avg. $(000)	No. (%)	Avg. $(000)
HOSPITAL	1,125	2,915,540	2,400	440 (.36)	3,621	406 (.33)	4,402	170 (.14)	1,584	140 (.12)	6,688	28 (.02)	230	37 (.03)	813
NURSING HOME	989	1,011,795	1,023	67 (.07)	1,200	174 (.18)	1,322	169 (.17)	544	565 (.57)	1,313	1 (.001)	10	9 (.009)	253
OTHER	210	383,798	1,828	24 (.11)	532	12 (.06)	1,751	42 (.20)	3,304	119 (.57)	2,892	9 (.04)	79	13 (.06)	1079
TOTAL PROJECTS	2,414	4,311,133	1,786	531 (.22)		592 (.25)		381 (.16)		824 (.34)		38 (.02)		59 (.02)	

between hospitals was not. In addition, some states received a fairly large number of poorly developed and clearly unacceptable nursing home proposals from real estate speculators. Finally, both nursing home associations and some agency staff stated that nursing homes are far less influential on state and area councils than are hospitals.

Even so, it seems clear that long term care is a growth industry which can be expected to account for an increasing proportion of total health care expenditures. New LTC beds were approved in much larger numbers (93.9% of 115,935 beds proposed) than new acute care beds (69.3% of 9,101 beds proposed). Based on Hill-Burton survey data, the additional beds approved by the 17 sample states amounted to 25% of their existing LTC beds. In contrast, the additional hospital beds approved amounted to only 2% of the existing beds.

Of all proposals to purchase equipment, 95.7% were approved; similarly 94.6% of all proposed additions of services were approved. The principal exceptions to these high approval rates for equipment and service proposals were proposals for X-ray and other scanner equipment, where the few denials were largely the result of several institutions' applying to purchase the same new equipment, (e.g., EMI scanners) with only one being approved. Discussions with agency staff indicated that their lack of criteria for most types of equipment and special services made it extremely difficult to deny these proposals. It should be noted that the projects on which these approval rates are based generally do not include the equipment purchases proposed as part of large new construction or renovation projects, since these proposals seldom identified equipment purchases separately, even though it was apparent from the proposal that new equipment was to be installed.

In summary, it appears that the most expensive form of health care—acute inpatient care—was being perpetuated and somewhat expanded, while at the same time long term and ambulatory facilities were being added to the health care system. This trend should be viewed with concern, if only because there is no evidence that this pattern of development reflects a conscious strategy based on a carefully developed vision of what the health care system should look like. For example, most agencies did not see long term care as a low-cost alternative to hospital care, but instead viewed the two types of care as largely unrelated. Thus, many agencies did not take into account hospital length of stay overall or length of stay for persons over 65 in considering long term care proposals or making long term care bed projections. Similarly, most agencies did not perceive ambulatory services in relation to inpatient care. Agency staff frequently reported that "we've finished our acute care plan and are now starting to work on our ambulatory care plan;" i.e., the two types of services were seen as independent of each other.

Effectiveness of CES Controls

It is apparent from the discussion thus far that, at least in the sample states and areas, the administration of CON and 1122 controls was flawed by inadequate plan development and deficiencies in review criteria and data resources. In the final analysis, however, the effectiveness of these controls must be determined on the basis of their success in preventing the development of unneeded health facilities and services. CON and 1122 agencies frequently argued that approval rates per se were not a reasonable measure of their effectiveness because, it was claimed, the agencies screened out or modified unneeded projects through various informal mechanisms prior to formal review. The tactics claimed by review agencies for discouraging unneeded proposals included negative agency response to provider inquiries, negotiation with providers before or during the review process, delaying unwanted applications through repeated requests for further information, and so on.

It may well be that such tactics significantly reduced the number of proposals which were formally reviewed and thus resulted in deceptively high approval rates; it was not possible to assess systematically the actual frequency of this behavior. However, whether or not CON and 1122 agencies successfully discouraged unneeded proposals, it seemed to us that a fair measure of agency effectiveness would be the net result of agency approvals in relation to their published need projections.

To apply this measure, we obtained the five-year Hill-Burton acute and long term bed projections for each sample state and area. When available, agency-developed bed projections were substituted for the Hill-Burton data. For example, the number of hospital beds approved during the survey period was then added to the number of existing hospital beds as shown in the need projection, and the percentage of projected bed need, represented by approved plus existing beds, was calculated.

Measurement of success in controlling non-bed investments was more difficult, as virtually no state or area agency had any need projections for ambulatory care, equipment, or special inpatient services. As a proxy measure, each state and area was ranked in terms of the percentage increase in existing hospital assets represented by all types of hospital projects approved during the survey period.

An analysis of performance against these measures by the 41 sample states and areas for which complete data could be obtained revealed that nearly 61% of the sample states and areas (25 of 41) had hospital beds in excess of 105% of their published need projection for five years hence at the beginning of the survey period. Fourteen (56%) of these approved additional beds, thus further increasing their overbedding; five other states became overbedded during the period studied as a result of the projects they approved. Thus, the addition of unneeded beds occurred in a total of 46% of the cases analyzed.

Only six states and areas began the period with more than 105% of the projected need for long term care beds. However, five of these approved still more beds and eight other jurisdictions approved additions to bed supply that made them overbedded. A total of 31% (13 of 41) states and areas appear to have failed to control excess LTC beds through CON or 1122 processes.

With respect to the third measure, an increase in hospital assets of 16% or more (estimated general economic growth plus inflation) was used as a standard. Only four state and four area agencies approved increases of this magnitude, but these increases were not systematically related to the per capita level of hospital assets in place prior to the survey period. These findings are relatively more encouraging than the effects of CON and 1122 controls on bed supply, although the long term cost implications of overbedding may be more serious.

These admittedly crude and limited measures of the effectiveness of CON and 1122 controls in preventing unnecessary capital expenditures present a somewhat unimpressive picture of the base on which PL 93-641 must build. At the same time, it is clear that many state and area agencies were performing effectively. In order to identify those aspects of CON and 1122 systems which were associated with superior performance and which should be strengthened nation-wide for implementation of the new law, both inspection of the data and, where feasible, simple bivariate correlations and *chi*-square analyses were used to determine the relationship between system variables and effectiveness.

Factors Associated with Effectiveness

Six states—New York, Ohio, Indiana, Connecticut, Michigan, and Georgia—consistently ranked in the top five in controlling hospital beds and assets. It is significant that some form of prospective rate controls for hospitals—administered by either the state or Blue Cross—is in place in all of these states except Georgia. Officials in these states expressed the view that, by placing provider institutions at risk with respect to future revenues, rate controls force these institutions to weigh more carefully the economic and financial feasiblity of capital projects.

In addition to the presence of rate controls, the states and areas that appeared most effective in administering facility and service controls shared certain other characteristics, including:

1. A somewhat greater expressed commitment to cost containment as the primary objective of facility and service regulation.

2. Comparatively high salaries and low turnover among state agency directors. (Rather surprisingly, the educational/professional background of agency directors and their staff was not found to be systematically related to performance.)

3. Assignment of the CON or 1122 control function to the Hill-Burton agency or a special unit created to administer these controls; states with CHP agencies administering controls generally appeared less effective than others.

4. Well-developed review criteria, covering a broad range of facilities and services.

The ability of CON or 1122 controls to enforce need projections also varied in relationship to the existing supply of health facilities, measured in terms of hospital beds/1,000 population. High bed ratios generally meant less effective controls, which suggests that whatever factors stimulated the development of a generous supply of hospital beds were still at work.

Agency and provider officials expressed the view that a key factor in overbedding is the reimbursement policies of third-party payors which, because they remove the financial risk of low occupancy, make hospitals in particular vulnerable to pressures to construct larger and more elaborate facilities. However, at the state level, there existed almost no communication or cooperation between review agencies and state agencies purchasing health services (e.g., Medicaid) or regulating third party payors (i.e., insurance commissions) except in one or two states where such cooperation is a routine feature of formal rate regulation.

At the area level, health planning and regulation was most effective where local industry actively supported and participated in these efforts; however, industry participation appeared to be more a result of civic pride than of informed concern about rising employee benefit costs. Thus, it is not clear whether industry involvement can be stimulated in other communities on the basis of enlightened self-interest.

EFFICIENCY AND FAIRNESS OF THE REVIEW PROCESS

To be truly effective instruments of public policy, CON controls must produce certain outcomes; in addition, they must achieve these outcomes in a manner that is efficient and fair to those affected. However, efficiency is an elusive concept in health care facility and service regulation where there are no agreed-on means of defining or measuring effectiveness. A similar problem exists with respect to assessing the fairness of reviews. Fairness, or justice, is not an absolute and by its very nature implies a weighing and balancing of competing interests and values. This balancing process is complicated in CON reviews by the lack of a consensus as to the "public good." Therefore, to assess efficiency and fairness, it is necessary to fall back on "process measures" and common sense. With these as criteria, several conclusions were possible and are discussed below.

Efficiency of CON and 1122 Reviews

The average elapsed time from initial submission of a project application to the final CON or 1122 decision ranged from a low of 58 days (Kansas) to a high of 178 days (New York). Variations in the duration of reviews—and therefore, presumably, the cost of these reviews, at least to providers—did not appear to be directly related to effectiveness. Instead, the duration of reviews was a result of three factors:

1. *Requests for information*, after receipt of an initial application, were probably the single most important factor in determining the length of reviews. While the number of requests is in part a function of the degree of controversy surrounding a proposal, most appeared to result from unclear application requirements and poor provider planning.

2. *The number of review levels,* which varied from a low of two to a high of six for individual states. While not related to effectiveness, a greater number of review levels may indicate a more open process since it usually means results of review committees are used at both the state and area levels.

3. *Complexity of reviews,* that is, whether a proposal is large or small, for a hospital or a nursing home, etc. and, as a function of these variables, whether the review is substantive or nonsubstantive.

Section 1122 and nearly all CON programs had in common a number of organizational and procedural flaws which, in aggregate, substantially detracted from their efficiency and effectiveness:

1. *Applications* were poorly designed and confusing. As a result, provider time was wasted through requests for clarification and additional information, and reviews were frequently conducted without the benefit of critical provider data.

2. *Review procedures* failed effectively to differentiate between small, easily decided-on proposals and exceptionally large, complex proposals. Thus, nonsubstantive reviews required an average of 50 days to complete.

3. *The highly technical aspects* of reviews (e.g., financial analysis) were assigned redundantly to both the state and area levels instead of centralized to insure they were performed well. As a result, they tended to be performed poorly or not at all.

Effective solutions to these and similar problems had generally been developed and implemented by one or more states or areas, and could be readily adopted by the majority of states if they had adequate resources and leadership.

Fairness in CON and 1122 Reviews

There was clear evidence that a significant number of review agencies did not afford due process to proposed new entries into the local health service area, especially if the sponsor was a proprietary hospital chain. Proposals of all types submitted by proprietary sponsors had significantly lower approval rates than comparable proposals submitted by nonprofit institutions (Table 2-5); 30% of the sample state agencies freely expressed a bias against proprietary providers and 45% opposed hospital chains. Moreover, instances were observed in which agency latitude in areas such as requesting additional information was used to block proposals submitted by proprietary chains.

However, not all of the differences between the treatment of for-profit providers in CON or 1122 reviews and that accorded other types of providers was attributable to arbitrary discrimination. Proprietary hospital chains have been relatively active in recent years in constructing new facilities. Since the prevailing view in most areas is that hospital facilities are in oversupply, new facility proposals are less likely to be approved than are modernization of existing ones. In addition, proprietary hospitals are more likely to propose specialty hospitals which, depending on one's view, represent either desirable regionalization of services or a threat to the "full service" hospital, which many feel is the keystone of a balanced community health care system. Most health planning and review agencies tended to support full service hospitals. Finally, at least a few proprietary hospital and nursing home chains had clearly been irresponsible. For example, one hospital chain retained an attorney to sue an area agency before it had even notified the agency of its intention to submit a proposal for a new facility, which it turned out not to be able to finance. In another state, a nursing home chain sought 26 CONs, obtained 19, began construction in only three cases, and eventually allowed all 19 certificates to expire due to lack of financing.

However, even if it is granted that expansionary health care corporations have been moving against trends in the health industry and in the process have sometimes acted irresponsibly, interviews with review agencies confirmed that strong biases against for-profit providers did exist. Further, these biases affected the manner in which agencies exercised their discretionary powers to request additional information, discourage proposals from being submitted, present data in public hearings and, of course, arrive at their final determination.

THE HIDDEN COSTS OF CES CONTROLS

Economists and, more recently, government officials have expressed deep concern that government regulation of industries such as air transportation and interstate trucking has created or protected gross inefficiencies resulting in price levels in these industries that are substantially higher than would exist under free market conditions. The difference between actual prices in these industries and the lower prices that would exist without regulation amounts to a hidden cost which must be taken into account when weighing the costs and benefits of regulation.

Health care regulation, particularly the regulation of capital expenditures, is thought by some to exact the same sort of hidden cost through intervention in decisions that otherwise would be made in response to market forces. The study findings and conclusions with respect to three types of hidden costs are discussed in this section:

1. protecting inefficient providers;
2. discouraging innovation;
3. constraining the development of national and regional medical centers.

Protecting Inefficient Providers

On balance, CON controls as administered during the survey period did appear to protect inefficient providers from competition. Review agencies generally focused on holding total supply to the level of projected need. In pursuing this goal, agencies typically did not take into account the relative efficiency of alternative health care providers because agency staff lacked the technical expertise required to do so. In addition, review agencies tended to oppose new entries to the health system that would "harm" existing institutions, in part because of the influence of these institutions, but also out of genuine concern for the stability and

TABLE 2-5
APPROVAL RATES BY OWNERSHIP OF INSTITUTION

	Completed Reviews	APPROVED		DENIED	
		N	%	N	%
FOR PROFIT	585	504	86	81	14
NONPROFIT	892	865	98	14	02
PUBLIC	298	286	97	9	03
TOTAL	1,775	1,655	93	104	07

quality of the health care system. Thus, in the majority of health service areas which already had an excess supply of acute inpatient facilities, potentially more efficient providers of these same services were barred from entering the market and competing with existing institutions.

However, having said this, it is important to say also that even if CON and 1122 agencies were more dedicated to efficiency and better able to distinguish among providers on this basis, it is not at all clear that a more efficient delivery system would result. The "cost-plus" policies of third-party payors would support the continued operation of the most inefficient providers, making it highly unlikely that any benefits in the form of reduced health costs would accrue from agency support of increased competition. Review agencies knew this and, as a result, felt justified in not permitting or stimulating competition with inefficient providers.

Discouraging Innovation

The study produced no hard evidence that CON controls played a major role in blocking the development of innovations such as health maintenance organizations and free-standing ambulatory care facilities. All but 4 of the 163 projects of this type in the sample were approved. This, plus the fact that the very small number of these projects in the sample nearly all came from three states which had actively sponsored and subsidized their development, suggests that factors other than CON controls inhibited the development of these innovations.

However, there is evidence that innovations—if they ever are proposed in significant numbers—will be at a serious disadvantage in CON reviews if only because they are "new entries." In addition, there were isolated instances in which local review agencies clearly had blocked the development of innovative services such as surgicenters on the grounds that they would "harm" existing institutions.

Constraining the Development of National Medical Centers

In theory, review decisions guided solely by state and local health plans could retard the development of medical centers which provide highly specialized services on region-wide and nation-wide bases. To determine the actual effect of current controls on such institutions, it was necessary to rely on discussions with review agencies, provider associations, and, in a few cases, officials of such institutions. These discussions suggest that CON and 1122 controls presented no serious obstacle to the capital expenditure and service development plans of regional and national medical centers. On the contrary, these institutions appeared to be virtually exempt from effective review and control by existing agencies, so great is their prestige and the influence of their supporters.

At the same time, there is reason to believe that in at least some states and areas, the immunity from controls that has thus far been enjoyed by regional and national health centers may be coming to an end, especially in the case of medical schools. Both review agencies and the local provider communities appeared to be somewhat resentful of what they perceived as the high-handed behavior of some national and regional medical centers. This is particularly true with respect to teaching hospitals, which, it is claimed, expand more in response to increases in student population than health care needs and which attempt to recover teaching costs through patient service charges, thereby driving up area health expenditures.

CONCLUSIONS

It seems clear from the available evidence that, as administered in 1974-75, health care capital expenditure and service controls did not perform effectively in preventing unnecessary capital investment in health facilities and services and thus would not be likely to result in the containment of health costs. In the first place, the effect of provider proposals on health costs was seldom a major factor in area and state decisions on such proposals. Second, controls did not appear in many cases to limit the creation of new beds and services to the predefined levels of need, which are generally conceded to be fairly generous. Finally, the types of investments that were permitted under these controls did not presage the sorts of changes in the mix of health care facilities and services that are thought to be necessary to make the health care delivery system more cost effective, nor is there any evidence that review decisions were made based on consideration of the trade-offs between various types of care.

However, when evaluating public policy—in this case, the federal policy that supports CON controls as a means of limiting unnecessary capital investment and thereby containing health costs—it is essential to distinguish between the limitations that are inherent in the policy itself and those that result from the manner in which the policy is implemented. A number of states and areas had achieved at least relative success in limiting unneeded capital investment. Moreover, these states differed from the others in that they tended to have well-developed need projections, review criteria, and data resources. These factors can be replicated in other states and areas and, presumably, will lead to more effective regulation once they are in place. Even more encouraging, with a few key exceptions, there do not appear to be any major technological barriers to developing the needed review tools.

However, even where controls exist and have been in place for some time, state and local commitment and management capacity are crucial in determining whether the tools necessary for effective CON regulation are developed and used, and the deficiencies that existed in these areas were serious and widespread. Historically, federal sponsorship of state and area health planning has stopped short of mandating or even guiding the development of goals and priorities for the cost, quality, or organization of the health care system. While there is a great deal of logic to this approach—the federal government has neither the means nor the mandate to shape local health care systems—one consequence is that state and area health planning and CON regulation have not been responsive to the federal interest in containing health costs.

Here again, there is cause to be somewhat optimistic that PL 93-641 may signal some change in the latitude permitted states and areas in health planning by calling for review of their plans in relation to national guidelines and priorities and by mandating periodic HEW assessment of state and area performance. The performance standards and agency assessment program developed for state and area CHP agencies appeared to have resulted in marked improvements in the agencies we visited. The Sec. 1122 program, which increased both the authority and resources of state and area agencies, helped sustain these improvements, as did the increases in 314 funding that occurred at about the same time (although the additional federal funds were used, in part, to replace state and local funds). This suggests that additional improvements should be expected as a result of the further increases in funds and tighter performance standards expected to result from PL 93-641.

However, there is an important lesson to be learned from the pattern of agency goals and performance that we observed. The mandate of state and area health planning and regulatory agencies is too large to be performed well in all respects in the short term. Under these circumstances, federal priorities (e.g., cost containment and development of a more cost effective delivery system) will be served only if they are clearly articulated and translated into specific objectives and requirements that agencies must meet in the near term. Thus, if it is important to federal policy aims that expansion of acute inpatient services be limited and that alternatives to these high cost services be developed, federal guidelines and performance standards must clearly require that priority be given to developing plans and criteria in these areas. If this is not done, there is every reason to believe that, five years from now, a substantial number of HSAs and state agencies will not have gotten around to developing specific need projections and review criteria applicable to the majority of the new capital projects in their jurisdiction because they are still struggling to define all encompassing health goals and to "build credibility" with providers and the public.

The social and political barriers to a more cost-effective health care system present an even more serious problem. It is now unthinkable for most states or area-wide agencies to take action to close or significantly to reduce services in a community hospital or medical center. Existing hospitals, whether religious or secular, can always draw on a culturally engrained fund of emotion and good will to support their continuation. While greater efforts to increase community awareness of the cost implications of excess health facilities will help counter this response, it is not reasonable to expect that CON controls and agencies can, by themselves, resist the pressure to expand inpatient facilities.

The most promising solution to this problem appears to be a health regulatory system that combines CON controls and rate review systems; on every measure of effectiveness relating to hospital beds and assets, the most effective states had either state rate review or Blue Cross prospective payment systems. A major reason, according to state officials, is that these rate controls prevent the accumulation of cash reserves that stimu- .late investment planning and place providers at risk for unwise investment decisions.

These same officials argue that it is better public policy to use reimbursement controls to close or reduce uneconomic facilities and services. In denying a rate increase or imposing fiscal sanctions for low utilization, the state leaves with the individual provider institution the initiative and responsibility for deciding how to adjust the scope of its operations in response to projected revenues. If, on the other hand, the state attempts to direct the closing or consolidation of services or make such action a condition for approval of CES proposals, the state inevitably ends up substituting its judgment for that of the individual institution in deciding what specific changes to make and how. State officials also pointed out that denying a request for a rate increase is obviously less likely to provoke·public opposition than denying permission to construct or modernize a hospital.

In the event that some form of national health insurance becomes law, the need for rate regulation will be even more urgent. Leaving aside the issue of relative agency effectiveness, the important point is that even the most effective agencies have not had to face being charged with "denying everything." This will undoubtedly happen to any conscientious agency should the volume of proposals increase dramatically, and agencies may be tempted—or forced by public opinion—to retreat to "reasonable" rates of approval which have little to do with actual need. It is, therefore, all the more urgent that rate controls be adopted to remove incentives to providers to attempt expansion of capacity.

Both CON and rate regulation are essential and complementary. Rate review, without CON planning and regulation, runs the risk of causing a long term deterioration in the capital assets of the health care system as a result of short term "marginal cost" decisions. At the same time, even the best existing CON controls will tend to optimize health care supply around identified needs and technological developments and, by not weighing "marginal cost" considerations, will tend to price health care beyond our means. In order for federal policy aims in health to be met, it is imperative that the nation pursue a balanced health regulatory strategy.

Even without any fundamental changes in federal policy concerning rate controls, there is a great deal that can be done and has been done to make states and areas more aware of and concerned about health costs and generally to improve the performance of health planning and regulatory agencies. During the past year, the Bureau of Health Resources Planning and Development has actively proceeded to develop criteria, planning guidance, and informational materials which should help raise the overall capacity of states and HSAs to perform effectively. Finally, the fact that 47 of the 50 states have now had at least two years' experience in the use of CON or 1122 regulation in itself holds great promise for the rapid improvement of the health care capital expenditures and services control effort under PL 93-641.

Notes

1. Research reported in this chapter was conducted for the U.S. Department of Health, Education and Welfare under Contract No. HRA-106-74-183. The data, conclusions, and recommendations are those of Lewin & Associates and do not represent the position of HEW or its constituent agencies.

2. Illinois enacted its CON law after the sample was selected. It was treated as a "no control" state for purposes of the study, as the law was not implemented during the study period.

3. *Nationwide Survey of State Health Regulations.* Report prepared for the Department of Health, Education and Welfare under Contract No. HEW-05-73-212 by Lewin & Associates, 1974.

4. *The Certificate of Need Experience: An Early Assessment.* Report prepared for Department of Health, Education and Welfare under contract No. HSM 110-73-749 by Macro Systems, Inc., 1974.

5. The number of proposals reported on in this and other tables is less than the total number of 2,891 proposals studied because state files for some proposals were incomplete.

Chapter 3

Regulation of Health Facilities and Services under Public Law 93-641

Edward J. Hanley

For all practical purposes, the debate over whether there should be binding public regulation of health facilities and services came to an end with the enactment of PL 93-641. Also known as the National Health Planning and Resources Development Act of 1974, PL 93-641 requires that each state establish and administer a certificate of need program that meets federal standards and spells out directly or by reference much of what must be contained in the federal standards. At the same time, PL 93-641 does allow the state sufficient latitude to design a CON program that is responsive to the unique characteristics and requirements of its health care system and style of government.

The purpose of this chapter is to explain those provisions of PL 93-641 that pertain to CON regulation and examine the implications of this landmark legislation for states and health care institutions. The discussion is presented in three parts as follows:

1. *The Intent and Basic Provisions of PL 93-641* This first section presents a brief overview of PL 93-641, describes the CON and related provisions of the law, and discusses the apparent intent of Congress in adopting these provisions.

2. *Standards for CON Programs Under PL 93-641* This section discusses what is likely to be required of states and of providers under the CON and related provisions of PL 93-641, at least insofar as this can be determined in the absence of final federal regulations, which have not yet been issued. In particular, the discussion highlights those areas in which states have retained the greatest flexibility in designing their CON programs.

3. *Implementation Issues and Problems* This final section returns to the research findings presented in Chapter two concerning the effectiveness of CON regulation to raise several major questions that must

eventually be confronted by both state regulators and provider institutions under the regulatory framework established by PL 93-641.

THE INTENT AND BASIC PROVISIONS OF PL 93-641

PL 93-641 is the product of long months of committee hearings and floor debate in both houses of Congress. This deliberative process was itself the outgrowth of numerous research and evaluation studies documenting the inability of existing federal and state policies to control the development of excess health facilities and services and the associated increases in health costs. In fact, as early as 1972, the Congress found that federal and state practices in reimbursing health care institutions for services provided to persons covered by the Medicare or Medicaid programs were a major cause of overinvestment and inflation in the health industry. This finding was the basis for enactment of the Section 1122 review program as part of the 1972 Amendments to the Social Security Act.

Unfortunately for those trying to understand and apply PL 93-641, the final form of the legislation does not reflect the effort actually invested by the various committees in developing this legislation. The bill finally enacted by Congress was drafted and passed in a rush during the final days of the first session of the Ninety-third Congress, which was trying to dig out of the enormous backlog created by the Watergate affair. As a result, PL 93-641 is replete with technical flaws and internal inconsistencies. Moreover, important substantive changes were introduced in the closing days of the debate, including amendments that eliminated the controversial requirements for state-administered rate controls and recertification of health care institutions and others that strengthened the role of state and local general-purpose governments and elected officials. Time apparently did not permit smooth integration of these changes into the final legislation.

In part because the bill is poorly drafted and unclear or contradictory in defining key requirements and responsibilities, no fully satisfactory, official synopsis of PL 93-641 has yet been published. This discussion does not presume to fill this void; rather, the intent is merely to provide a broad overview of PL 93-641 in its entirety and describe those provisions relating to regulation of health facilities and services.

It is quite clear from the preamble to PL 93-641 that by enacting this legislation, Congress intended first, to reaffirm that equal access to quality health care is a priority of the federal government and second, to clarify and strengthen the network of local, state, and federal programs responsible for achieving this priority. More specifically, the law does the following:

It establishes a single, unitary network of state and regional agencies responsible for all health planning, resource development and facility and service review functions to replace the existing patchwork of largely federally sponsored state and area-wide health planning and resource development programs. Thus, the law eliminates state and area health planning agencies authorized by Sections 314(a) and (b) of the Public Health Service Act, the Experimental Health Systems Development programs, and the Regional Medical Programs. In place of this tangle of overlapping agencies and programs, PL 93-641 establishes a single network consisting of health systems agencies at the area level and a State Health Planning and Development (SHPD) agency overseen by a State Health Coordinating Council (SHCC). While certain of the functions assigned to states by PL 93-641 may be delegated to agencies other than the SHPD agency, these delegations are subject to approval by the federal government and, in any case, do not relieve the SHCC and the SHPD agency of ultimate accountability for state level health planning and resources development functions.

To insure public participation at both the area and state levels, the law sets strict requirements for consumer membership in the HSA governing boards and the SHCC. In addition, to insure that state health planning and resource development activities are responsive to local health planning, HSAs are given control over the appointment of over 50% of the SHCC members.

It recasts federal programs providing capital financing for medical facilities to give greater emphasis to noninstitutional health care and increased responsiveness to local priorities. Title XVI of PL 93-641 replaces the Hill-Burton program with a new program of capital financing that has two components:

1. State-administered construction and modernization financing that is allocated to priorities established by the SHCC in consultation with the HSAs as well as the state agency. The priorities that must be adhered to in allocating these monies are strongly biased in favor of outpatient care and correcting maldistribution problems.

2. Locally administered resource development funds intended for use as seed money to launch new and innovative health services and delivery systems.

It mandates that all states establish binding controls on the development of institutional health facilities and services and voluntary recertification of these same facilities and services at five-year intervals. As mentioned at the outset of this chapter, PL 93-641 requires that all states adopt CON programs that regulate the development of new institutional health facilities and services and that such programs meet federal standards for coverage, public participation, and due process. Moreover, a section of the law which is often overlooked by states and providers—Section 1522(b)(7)(B)—provides that states must require regular statistical and other reports by all health care providers doing business in the state. This provision should bring to an early end the debate that has gone on for many years, at least in states with no CON programs, about the desirability and legality of requiring hospitals and other health care institutions to make regular reports on capacity, utilization, and cost data.

The second, voluntary review requirement established by PL 93-641 is a mandate that each HSA and state review and report publicly on the "appropriateness" of all existing institutional health facilities and services at least once every five years. This provision is what finally resulted from strong efforts by some in the Congress to establish a formal recertification process in which facilities and services that were deemed appropriate would be phased out of existence. It remains to be seen what effect the voluntary appropriateness review process will have; some third-party reimbursement agencies have already expressed interest in denying coverage to facilities and services adjudged to be "inappropriate" by the state.

It requires that the federal government and specifically HEW monitor and enforce standards of performance for area and state health planners and regulators. The Congress appears to be saying quite clearly that, with federal health expenditures now well in excess of $20 billion annually, nearly 30% of total health expenditures, the federal government can no longer afford a laissez-faire approach to state and local efforts to plan and regulate health resource development. It remains to be seen whether and how HEW will respond to this mandate; however, it seems likely that an even stronger incentive for state action is the fact that health care expenditures by state and local governments approximate those of the federal government both in absolute terms and in their rate of increase. In the event that the health planning and regulatory framework established by PL 93-641 fails to contain health cost increases, it can be predicted that states will move to more direct methods of health cost containment, namely regulation of provider rates.

STANDARDS FOR CON PROGRAMS UNDER PL 93-641

PL 93-641 requires that each state agency administer a certificate of need program which applies to new institutional health services proposed to be developed or offered within the state and which is satisfactory to the Secretary. The precise coverage, procedures, and sanctions required in order for a CON program to be deemed satisfactory are discussed in subsequent sections; however, it is the expressed view of Congress that the major purpose of state CON programs must be to prevent the construction or other development of unnecessary and inappropriate health care facilities and services. Recognizing this, the Secretary of HEW has made it clear in the proposed regulations for implementing PL 93-641 that only CON programs that clearly accomplish this will be deemed satisfactory.

In addition to establishing the legal and administrative capacity to achieve this basic purpose, each state must satisfy certain general requirements in developing and administering its CON program:

- *Procedures and Criteria.* In administering the CON program, the state agency must follow procedures and apply criteria that have been developed and published in accordance with regulations of the Secretary of HEW. The specific requirements of the law in this respect are outlined below.

- *Enforcement.* An essential feature of each state CON program must be that it "provide that only those [health] services, facilities and organizations found to be needed shall be offered or developed in the state." The specific sanctions that seem likely to satisfy the federal government at least initially are outlined below; the adequacy of any sanction or set of sanctions will ultimately be determined by the federal government based on the experience of states in applying them.

- *Role of Health Systems Agencies and the Public.* PL 93-641 also specifies that, in administering the CON program, state agencies shall consider the recommendations of HSAs and make explicit provisions for broad public participation in the review process. Specific provisions of the law pertaining to the role of HSAs and the public in CON reviews are also discussed below.

The deadline for state compliance with the CON provisions of PL 93-641 is one of those areas in which the law is less than clear. Section 1523(b)(2) of the law provides that the CON requirement goes into force upon the expiration of "the first regular session of the (state) legislature ... which begins after the date of enactment" of PL 93-641. However, in part since final federal regulations interpreting the CON requirement have not yet been issued, few, if any, states have moved to comply with this deadline, which in nearly all cases has now expired.

A more realistic deadline, and one which the federal government might be expected to enforce, can be derived from other provisions of the law pertaining to federal designation of a state health planning and resources development agency as fully satisfying all aspects of PL 93-641. Section

1521(d) of the law provides that states have until the "expiration of the fourth fiscal year which begins after the calendar year" in which PL 93-641 is enacted to come into compliance with the full terms and conditions of the law. Failure to meet this deadline—which falls on September 30, 1980—would mean that the state and all institutions within the state would be barred from receiving federal monies under the Public Health Service Act, the Comprehensive Alcohol Abuse and Alcoholism Prevention Treatment and Rehabilitation Act of 1970, and the Community Mental Health Centers Act. The loss of these monies would have a devastating effect on state and local public health agencies, medical centers and social services programs; thus, it seems likely that this deadline, if enforced by the federal government, will be adhered to by the states.

For the time being at least, Congress has extended both the authority and funding for reviews of proposed capital expenditures under Section 1122 of the Social Security Act. Once universal state CON programs are in place, the Section 1122 program may well be eliminated; however, there are many who argue that the Sec. 1122 enforcement mechanism, which relies on federal audits and denial of reimbursement, should be retained under any circumstances. In the short term, it is expected that states will coordinate and eventually fully integrate the administration of CON programs and their reviews under Section 1122. The proposed federal regulations governing state agency organization and functions require that both review activities be administered by the same agency of state government, whether that be the designated state agency or another agency selected by the governor and approved by the Secretary. In addition, to facilitate the integration of CON and Section 1122 reviews, the proposed federal regulations governing both review programs have been made identical in all possible respects. Thus, for example, the review procedures previously required under Section 1122 are being revised to correspond to the requirements of PL 93-641; similarly, "health care facility" and "health maintenance organization"—the entities subject to review—are being defined identically by both review programs.

Section 1122 will, nonetheless, remain distinct from state CON programs in one important respect. The Section 1122 authority applies only to changes in facilities and services which involve a capital expenditure, whereas PL 93-641 requires that CON coverage extend to certain service changes whether or not a capital expenditure is involved.

The remainder of this section of the chapter describes the requirements and standards set by PL 93-641 regarding three aspects of state CON programs:

- Coverage

- Enforcement
- Review procedures and criteria

Coverage

The coverage mandated by PL 93-641 for state CON programs includes all "new institutional health services" that are proposed to be offered or developed in or through a health facility or health maintenance organization, and certain predevelopment activities associated with offering or developing such services. A health care facility or organization is considered to be "offering" specific health services when it holds itself out as capable of providing such services. "Developing" a service means undertaking an activity or incurring a financial obligation (as defined under applicable state law) which is related to or will result in new services being offered. The two types of covered items—new institutional health services and predevelopment activities—are examined separately below.

New Institutional Health Services

The meaning of the term "new institutional health services" is perhaps best understood if it is conceived of as establishing a two-part test for determining whether a proposed expenditure or service change is subject to review. The first part of the test is to determine whether the proposed new institutional health service is to be offered in or through a "health care facility" or "HMO" as defined by PL 93-641. Second, it is necessary to determine whether the proposed expenditure or change leads up to or will result in a "new" service being offered by the facility or organization in question. The requirements and standards established by PL 93-641 concerning both aspects of this two-part test are outlined below.

Facilities and Organizations Subject to Review. With certain specific exceptions, Section 1531(5) of PL 93-641 mandates coverage of the health care facilities and HMOs encompassed by the definitions set forth in regulations prescribed under Section 1122 of the Social Security Act (42 CFR, Part 100). "Health care facilities" are defined as including:

- Hospitals, including psychiatric and tuberculosis hospitals
- Skilled nursing and intermediate care facilities
- Kidney disease treatment centers, including free-standing hemodialysis units
- Ambulatory surgical facilities

A "Health Maintenance Organization" (HMO) is defined as a public or private organization, organized under the laws of any state, which has three basic characteristics:

- It provides or makes available to enrolled participants at least the following health care services: usual physician services, hospitalization, laboratory, X-ray, emergency, and preventive services and out-of-area coverage.
- It is compensated, except for copayments, on a predetermined periodic rate basis.
- It provibes physician services primarily through physicians who are either direct employees or partners or with whom specific prior arrangements have been made.

Home health agencies, outpatient physical therapy facilities and organized ambulatory care facilities (with the exception of ambulatory surgical facilities), while covered by Section 1122, are not "institutional" health services and, thus, need not be covered by state CON programs to satisfy PL 93-641. In addition, Christian Science sanatoriums operated or listed and certified by the First Church of Christ Scientist, Boston, Massachusetts, are specifically exempted from the required federal coverage. In all cases, of course, states are free to extend CON coverage to facilities and services exempted by the federal law.

Expenditures and Service Changes Subject to Review. A health care facility or HMO subject to state CON programs is considered to be proposing the development or offering of a "new" institutional health service when one of four elements is present:

- *New facility or organization.* The construction, development, or any other form of establishment of a new health care facility or HMO is subject to review.
- *Capital expenditure in excess of $150,000.* Proposed federal regulations for state CON programs now under review state that any capital expenditure in excess of $150,000 made by or on behalf of a covered health care facility or HMO is subject to review, whether or not patient care is directly affected. Thus, expenditures for heating and air conditioning equipment, parking lots, office buildings, land acquisition, and similar nonpatient care capital assets must be covered by state CON programs. Expenditures required to correct licensure and other code violations must also be covered, although provisions may be made for an expeditious review under certain circumstances, such as when patient health and safety are threatened.
- *Changes in existing bed structure.* Coverage is required of any change in existing bed complement through the addition, relocation, or conversion of one or more beds. However, states will be permitted to exercise discretion in making provisions for emergency, temporary, or seasonal changes in bed complement. Similarly,

states may establish review procedures that permit expeditious administrative treatment of small changes in bed complement so long as there are clearly defined thresholds and other criteria for determining when a change is "minor," and safeguards to prevent providers from escaping a full review of major changes in bed structure by making small incremental changes over time.

PL 93-641 does not require that state CON programs cover reductions in bed complement. However, a number of states have chosen to regulate this form of change in bed structure and such coverage is not precluded by the federal law.

Addition of new services. Addition of any health service not previously provided by a covered health care facility or organization is subject to review whether or not a capital expenditure is involved. The review of new services not involving a capital expenditure is required to comply with the expressed intent of Congress that "only those services. . . found to be needed. . . shall be offered or developed in the State" [Section 1523(a)(4)(B)]. However, it is not the intent of Congress that this requirement result in unnecessarily obtrusive involvement in minor staff and program changes by health care institutions.

The term "health services" means clinically related (i.e., diagnostic, curative or rehabilitative) services and includes alcohol, drug abuse, and mental health services. It will be up to each state to expand upon and clarify the definition of "new service" in a manner that makes sense in relation to such factors as existing state codes governing the licensure of health care facilities and services and in a way that provides for efficient administration of its CON program.

Predevelopment Activity

Section 1523(a)(4)(B) of PL 93-641 also requires that a CON program provide for review and determination of need prior to the time substantial expenditures are undertaken in preparation for the offering or development of a new institutional health service. HEW has proposed that the term "substantial" be defined as meaning any amount in excess of $150,000 (or any lesser amount that a state may choose). Therefore, state CON programs must specifically require review and approval of any proposed expenditure in excess of $150,000 for predevelopment activities.

There is nothing in PL 93-641 that precludes states from establishing a two stage CON process in which approval is first granted solely for predevelopment expenditures such as those for surveys, studies, and plans without authorizing actual development or offering of a new institutional health service. Several states now employ this two-stage approach in cases involving large capital projects, since the development of detailed plans sufficient to permit a full assessment of the need for and financial feasibility of such projects will often, by itself, exceed any reasonable dollar threshold for CON review. The two-stage approach permits the state to authorize investment in detailed planning for what, in concept, appears to be a worthy project without commitment itself to final approval until the sponsor provides full details. Similarly, in some instances this approach may protect providers by enabling them to seek approval for a basic service concept before risking large sums on predevelopment activities.

Enforcement

PL 93-641 is quite straightforward with respect to enforcement of state CON programs; Section 1523(a)(4)(B) states that "such programs shall . . . provide that only those services, facilities, and organizations found to be needed shall be offered or developed in the State." More specifically, in order to be judged satisfactory by the secretary, a state CON program must insure that CONs are granted only to new institutional health services which the state has found to be needed and that new institutional health services shall be offered or developed within the state only if such services have been granted a CON.

In order to satisfy federal requirements with respect to enforcement, state CON programs must make explicit provisions for sanctions to be imposed on those who refuse to submit to CON reviews or elect to violate CON rulings. It is up to each state to select the sanction or combination of sanctions that is best suited to its own needs, so long as the practical effect of the sanctions chosen is to prevent the development or offering of new institutional health services without state approval. In the final analysis, the determination made by the federal government as to the adequacy of any particular sanction or set of sanctions will be based on the effectiveness of such sanctions as demonstrated by experience. In view of this, states should consider adopting a system to monitor the development of new services and facilities that have received CONs to insure that the terms and conditions of the certificate are being honored. For example, a large facility project might easily evolve over the course of its development until there are substantial changes not only in the total expenditure being made (which, if the increase is more than $150,000, should trigger a new CON review) but also in the level and mix of services to be offered by the completed project.

The type of provider reporting that would be necessary for such a monitoring system need not be either onerous or foreign to health care institutions. Comparable progress reporting has long been required by the Hill-Burton program and other similar federal and state programs to finance the development of health care facilities and services as well as by many state licensing agencies. Moreover, the data required in such reports should be no more than is routinely available to the sponsor of the new facility or service that is being developed. Monitoring based on periodic provider reports is a fairly common practice among states that already have CON programs and quite often is coupled with some form of site inspection, particularly in states that rely on denial of licensure to enforce CON decisions.

The types of sanctions now employed or being considered for state CON programs are discussed below in terms of their acceptability under PL 93-641.

Denial or Revocation of Operating License

Nearly all states require that health care facilities be licensed in order to operate. In determining whether denial or revocation of licensure is a suitable sanction, careful consideration should be given to the capacity of the licensure code to distinguish among services. In some states, the licensure code defines only broad categories of facilities such as "hospital," "nursing home," etc. In these states, it may be operationally difficult or impossible to use denial or revocation of the operating licensure as an effective sanction because appliiation of the sanction would mean closing the entire facility—a sanction so harsh that it seems unlikely to be applied effectively. For example, it could be difficult to justify or gain public support for withdrawing the operating license for an entire hospital merely because it has converted pediatric beds to general medical/surgical use, particularly if both categories of beds are encompassed by its operating license.

Civil or Criminal Penalties

Although now a part of many state CON and licensure programs, the potential weakness of civil and criminal penalties is that they can be so severe as to make it inconceivable that they would be applied to a non-profit community institution such as a hospital. Thus, if such penalties are selected as sanctions for a CON program, provisions should be made for flexibility in their application. Another potential drawback of this form of sanction is that such penalties can be imposed only after a violation has occurred.

Injunctive Relief

This sanction is also a part of many existing CON programs and, in many ways, is the most flexible and easiest to apply. However, states that elect to adopt this sanction should insure that the CON agency has ready access to the courts so that timely injunctive relief is a reality. It could become impractical in both an economic and political sense to enforce CON rulings if enforcement meant undoing an action already taken and resulted in great cost to a nonprofit community hospital or public institution. Moreover, if it appears that injunctive relief could not in fact be obtained in time to forestall the development or offering of services without state approval, this sanction might not be ruled acceptable by the federal government.

Denial of Reimbursement

A fourth type of sanction in which some states have expressed an interest is denial of reimbursement. One form of this sanction is used in the Section 1122 program which provides for denial of federal reimbursement for the portion of costs attributable to an unapproved capital expenditure. However, partial or even full denial or reimbursement by Medicaid and other third party payors under state control has a serious deficiency in the context of PL 93-641, in that it can only be applied after the fact of a capital expenditure and does not necessarily prevent unapproved services from being offered. PL 93-641 requires both that the expenditure not be permitted in the first place and that CON programs cover some service changes in which no capital expenditure is involved. Even if all third party reimbursement were denied, application of this sanction would still be after the fact and would allow for development and offering of new services aimed entirely at the private pay market. In light of these weaknesses, denial of reimbursement is not likely to satisfy federal standards unless it is used in conjunction with other types of sanctions.

Review Procedures and Criteria

Section 1532(a) of PL 93-641 requires that, in conducting reviews of proposed or existing health services, each state agency and HSA "follow procedures and apply criteria developed and published in accordance with [Federal] regulations." In broad terms, CON review procedures and criteria must satisfy federal requirements in two areas: (1) the manner in which they are adopted and published and (2) their substance.

Adoption of CON Review Procedures and Criteria

PL 93-641 mandates that, whatever the substance of the procedures and criteria that are adopted by state agencies and HSAs, these agencies must meet certain requirements pertaining to timing and public notice in both adopting and revising such procedures and criteria. The three principal requirements in this regard are:

- Each state agency and HSA must adopt review procedures and criteria that meet federal requirements not later than three months from the date of its designation as a state or area planning and review agency under the terms of PL 93-641.
- Before final adoption, state agencies and HSAs must give interested persons an opportunity to review and comment on the proposed procedures and criteria.
- Copies of adopted or revised review procedures and criteria must be circulated to all interested parties, and be available to anyone upon request.

Requirements for Review Procedures

The procedures adopted and followed by state agencies and HSAs in conducting CON reviews may vary in response to the purpose of a review or the type of proposal being reviewed, but must incorporate certain minimum provisions aimed primarily at insuring a review process that, while efficient, is fair and open to public scrutiny. PL 93-641 specifically requires the following:

Written notification of review. Written notification must be given to affected persons at the start of a review. Those given notice of the review must include, at a minimum, the sponsor of the proposal, all institutional health service providers in the area, and the public to be served by the proposed services. Written notification to the public may be made through general circulation newspapers; other affected parties must be notified by mail.

Schedule for reviews. The minimum requirements of PL 93-641 concerning the schedule for state CON and NIH reviews can be summarized as follows:

- To the extent practicable, all CON reviews must be completed 90 days from the date of notification of the beginning of a review. If a review period is to exceed 90 days, criteria must have been adopted for determining when it is not practicable to complete a review within 90 days.
- State CON review schedules must set forth a period within which HSA recommendations are to be provided and such period may not be less than 60 days from the start of the review except by written consent of the HSA.

These requirements for review schedules should not be unduly restrictive in the sense of precluding full and effective consideration even in large, complex CON proposals. Thus, for example, the 60-day period required for HSA review should be sufficient in all but a very few cases based on the documented experience of area agencies under Section 1122. Moreover, the law in effect permits states to exceed the 90 day limit whenever the state deems it necessary, so long as the ground rules authorizing longer reviews are published in advance. It is also assumed that state agencies and HSAs will devise arrangements for speedy consideration of emergency and nonsubstantive applications, despite the 60-day period mandated for HSA reviews.

Submission of information. State CON programs must both explicitly authorize the state agency to require persons subject to reviews to submit to the agency such information as the agency determines is needed to conduct the review and prescribe and publish these information requirements in advance. While not required to do so by federal law or regulation, states may wish to specify the source or sources to be used in compiling certain basic information such as population projections, existing health service or facility supply and utilization data, which are required in CON applications. Specifying sources in this manner—if provision is made for the applicant to argue in favor of using a source other than that specified—has two advantages. First, it informs potential applicants in advance of the data considered by the reviewing agency to be authoritative in determininl the need for a new institutional health service, and second, it contributes to efficiency by decreasing the need to request additional information from applicants in the course of reviews.

Submission of periodic reports. In addition to requiring that state agencies be empowered to prescribe application requirements, the law mandates that provisions be made for periodic reports from providers concerning the development of proposals subject to review. The form and content of such periodic reports may be determined by each state. The purpose of this requirement is to assure that state agencies and HSAs have access to information about the plans of health care providers to develop or offer new institutional health services while these plans are still in the formative stage. Possession of this information should afford these agencies the opportunity—before formal applications are submitted—to seek coordination both among providers and between provider plans and the state and area health plans and priorities. In addition, such information will permit state agencies and HSAs better to schedule project review resources and workload.

Written findings. At the completion of state CON reviews, written findings must be prepared that state the basis for the decision or recommendation made. These written findings must be sent to the sponsor of the proposal, to the affected HSA (in the case of findings by the state agency), and to anyone else upon request. States have considerable latitude in defining what must be contained in the written findings; however, the experience to date under Section 1122 and existing state CON programs indicates that there are benefits in terms of equity and public relations in clearly summarizing the basis for each decision. Moreover, there is some evidence that states that do publish a summary of the findings that underlie CON and Section 1122 decisions are less vulnerable to reversal upon appeal.

Notification of review status and outcome. Upon request, state agencies and HSAs are required to provide to those subject to review information concerning findings made in the course of the review, the status of the review itself, and any other appropriate information. States and HSAs are free to place reasonable limits on what is "appropriate" so long as the procedures published by review agencies make clear the obligation of the agency to give notice of review status and outcome and do not define limits on the information to be provided that violate the provisions or intent of PL 93-641.

Public hearings. The review procedures adopted for state CON programs and NIH reviews must provide for public hearings under two sets of circumstances:

- *In the course of a review.* A public hearing must be held in the course of a review at the request of any person "directly affected" by the proposal to develop or offer a new institutional health service. States may elect to establish CON procedures which provide for public hearings to be held either by both the state agency and the HSA, or by the HSA only. The original notice of the start of the review must inform those affected when requests for such a public hearing may be made and when a hearing is scheduled. In the course of the hearing, any person attending must be permitted to give testimony, whether or not "directly affected" by the proposal.

- *To reconsider a review decision.* State CON programs must provide that, for good cause shown, any person may request a public hearing to reconsider a state agency decision. At a minimum, "good cause" is shown if the request:
  — presents significant, relevant information not previously considered by the state agency
  — demonstrates that significant changes have occurred in factors or circumstances relied upon by the state agency in reaching its decision
  — demonstrates that the state agency has materially failed to follow its adopted review procedures.

States may, of course, define additional circumstances in which "good cause" will be deemed to have been shown. In addition, states may establish reasonable time limits for filing appeals— perhaps 30 to 60 days following notice of a decision.

The importance of written, published review procedures and findings becomes obvious when considered in light of the requirements for reconsideration hearings. Due process is weakened if procedures or findings are unclear since this can make it difficult to determine whether a hearing is required. Moreover, state agencies are vulnerable to reconsideration hearings on the grounds of new information if the findings published to support a decision are incomplete or unclear.

Appeals hearings. State CON programs must provide for formal appeals hearings if requested by an HSA when a state agency makes a decision that is inconsistent with the HSA's recommendation, or by the sponsor of a proposal that has been denied a CON. The appeals mechanisms for both HSAs and sponsors must provide for review by an agency of state government (other than the state agency) designated by the governor, and satisfy applicable state laws governing administrative hearings. The reviewing agency may support or overturn the state agency or remand the matter back to the state agency for further action. Except where remanded, the decision at the appeal level is final, short of adjudication in court.

In the past, some state CON programs have used appeals mechanisms that have amounted to little more than appeal to the next level of the health department—thus asking an agency to review its own actions. Such mechanisms will not meet the requirements of PL 93-641. Beyond this, the chief problem experienced by states in conducting appeals has been the use of hearing officers not well grounded in proper procedure or the particular ground rules of the CON or Section 1122 programs. States would be well advised to be thoughtful in designating the reviewing agency and to invest some effort to insure a cadre of well-prepared hearing officers. Experience suggests that the consequences of not doing so are either that the CON program is weakened or that the state is tied up in expensive litigation.

Decisions that conflict with HSA plans. In the event that a final decision rendered by the state agency (or, in the case of appeal hearings, by the appeal agency) is inconsistent with the goals and priorities set forth in the applicable area health plan, the agency rendering that decision is required to submit to that HSA a detailed statement of the reasons for the inconsistency. The procedures adopted by the state agency for CON reviews must make explicit provision for submission of such a detailed statement and, further, must specify that it is the responsibility of the state agency to determine when a conflict exists and a statement is required.

In considering this provision, it is important to bear in mind that Section 1524(c)(2)(A) authorizes the Statewide Health Coordination Council (SHCC) to revise area health plans as necessary "to achieve appropriate coordination with . . . the other agencies which participate in the SHCC or to deal more effectively with Statewide health needs." Thus, basic differences between statewide goals and priorities and those of an individual HSA should ordinarily be resolved in the context of the health plan development process, and not in the course of individual CON reviews.

Regular reports of review activity. PL 93-641 mandates that state agencies and HSAs shall prepare and publish regular reports of the reviews conducted by the CON program, including the status of ongoing reviews and the outcomes of completed reviews. The federal government appears certain to define "regular" as at least annually and to require states and HSAs to provide certain basic data concerning the characteristics and outcomes of CON reviews for purposes of federal policy review and evaluation. It seems likely that most states will also assemble and periodically analyze such data for their own purposes as one means of understanding trends in the health system state-wide and assessing the achievements of their CON programs.

Public access to information. State CON procedures must incorporate provisions that make explicit the right of the general public to have access to all applications that are reviewed as well as all related written materials. Arrangements may be made to grant access under conditions that insure the integrity of the files and assess reasonable fees for reproduction; however, such arrangements may not take a form that makes access unduly difficult or prohibitively expensive.

Letters of intent. Provisions must be made in review procedures to require the submission of letters of intent in the case of projects that will entail construction activities. Letters of intent must be submitted at the earliest possible date in the planning of such projects and in such detail as states determine is necessary to determine the scope and nature of the projects involved.

The rationale for letters of intent is that they will inform the state agency and HSA about major projects that are under consideration although not yet at the stage at which formal application can be made. If alerted to such projects at an early stage, these agencies can better coordinate potentially conflicting projects, suggest design features that are consistent with state and area health plans, and, when appropriate, undertake needs-assessment and plan-development activities, alone or in concert with affected providers, to establish a sound basis for better coordinating and eventually reviewing the proposed construction projects.

Additionally, many state CON programs have experienced problems in reviewing large, complex hospital construction projects because the normal review period is not sufficient. Moreover, it has proved difficult to deny such a proposal once it reaches the formal application stage because, by that point, there has already been a sizable investment in predevelopment activities and, quite often, substantial community sentiment in favor of the project even if ill conceived. The early warning provided by the letter of intent, along with the requirement for review of predevelopment expenditures, is meant to assist agencies in overcoming these problems.

Criteria for Review

The statute does not in fact mandate specific criteria that must be applied to proposals for new institutional health services. Instead, it specifies areas in which criteria are to be developed and provides that criteria may vary "according to the purpose for which a review is being conducted or the type of health service being reviewed." The areas in which PL 93-641 requires that review criteria be established are:

- The relationship of the proposed health services to the applicable HSP and AIP
- The relationship of proposed services to the long-range development plan (if any) of the sponsoring institution
- Needs of the population to be served
- Availability of alternative, less costly or more effective methods of providing proposed services
- Immediate and long term financial feasiblity
- Relationship of proposed services to the existing health care system
- Availability of resources
- Relationship to ancillary or support services
- Special needs and circumstances of entities serving populations beyond the state or health service area
- Special needs and circumstances of HMOs
- Cost and impact of construction projects, including:
  — The cost and methods of the proposed construction
  — The probable impact on the cost of providing services by the sponsoring institution.

At this juncture, it appears that the federal role regarding specific review criteria will be limited to one of financing research and technical assistance activities in support of state and HSA efforts to develop criteria. Two other factors seem likely to play a more important role in determining the type of criteria that are developed and the progress made in developing them.

First, the propensity of the provider community to resort to litigation has been a major force behind efforts in some states to devise very specific, concrete review criteria. Where state courts have overturned CON decisions on the grounds that review criteria are arbitrary in their formulation or unclear in the way they have been applied, CON agencies typically respond in one of the following ways: they invest heavily in developing more defensible criteria or they become less forceful as regulators.

A second factor determining the direction taken in developing review criteria appears to be the position taken by state courts in defining the state's regulatory powers. In some states, the courts appear to be insisting that there must be concrete, predefined criteria applied in a complete straightforward objective fashion. In others, such as Massachusetts, the courts have ruled that the CON process is a delegated legislative function, and therefore it is entirely appropriate that value judgements play a part in CON decisions.

IMPLEMENTATION ISSUES AND PROBLEMS

As pointed out in Chapter two, a significant number of states, and now the federal government, have embraced the concept of CON regulation as a means of rationalizing the development of health resources and containing health cost increases without knowing for certain that this form of regulation will achieve these ends and without understanding the potential side effects or "hidden costs" of CON regulation. The research findings discussed in Chapter two, while they do not invalidate the basic concept of CON regulation, do suggest that there are a number of troublesome questions that must be addressed by federal and state officials as they go about implementing the planning-regulatory framework defined by PL 93-641. It may even turn out that the ultimate resolution of at least some of these questions will require amending the federal law.

The remainder of this chapter is devoted to a brief examination of the issues and problems pertaining to CON regulation that are likely to prove important in achieving the goals of PL 93-641.

Provider Cooperation and Support

The experience to date suggests that, except in the very few states prepared to invest large sums of money in staff and other resources, health planning and CON regulation will succeed only to the extent that they receive the cooperation and support of major provider institutions and organizations. At the area level, there have been no instances of successful planning and review without provider cooperation and support whether given voluntarily or as a result of coercion by local industry and financial leaders.

In states where the provider community elects to oppose aggressively the operation of CON controls through litigation and other means, it seems certain that the administration of the review process will be extremely difficult and, at least in the short term, ineffective. Area and state agencies will experience great difficulty in obtaining needed data and the expert counsel from the health professions that they require to develop sound, explicit review criteria. Moreover, once the planning-regulatory process becomes an adversary proceeding, there quite often follows a general deterioration of provider restraint in developing new facilities and services. In more than a few communities, this has led to a cycle of expansion and counter-expansion among individual institutions to the point that all are damaged by low utilization and a loss of community support.

One fact now seems clear—the provider community can make or break health planning and regulation in the near term; however, over the long haul, the providers will lose. The major industries in the U.S. have begun to realize what health cost inflation means in terms of higher fringe benefit costs, and nearly all states as well as the federal government are growing less tolerant of rising medical assistance budgets. Provider institutions can, if they choose, continue to win public support for individual expansion projects through appeals to community pride. However, the eventual consequences of doing so appear certain to be a loss of political and financial support and eventual deterioration in their financial base.

The Demand for Rate Controls

The research findings discussed in Chapter two tend to support the argument that an effective health cost containment strategy must include direct prospective controls on provider reimbursement. Moreover, it is now quite clear that enactment of national health insurance legislation will carry with it rate regulation, probably administered by the state under federal supervision. Even if national health insurance is deferred for several more years, the probability that universal CON regulation will fail to contain health cost increases means that pressure will grow for state-initiated rate controls. The experience of those few states that now regulate provider reimbursement indicates that development of a satisfactory rate-setting process requires at least two years. States would be well advised to consider following the example of Arizona and begin a voluntary rate review process so that the extremely difficult technical questions and value judgements can be worked out in a nonthreatening atmosphere.

The Fate of Innovation in a Regulated Health Industry

Just at the time when direct regulation of health capital investment and service development has become the law of the land, many of the same researchers, economists, and consumer advocates who have long criticized the development of unneeded health facilities and services are now expressing deep concern that CON regulation will impede the development of HMOs, free-standing ambulatory care facilities and other, lower-cost alternatives to our present hospital-based health care system. The basis for their concerns has two components. First, any regulation of capital investment and service development in the health industry obviously will weigh heavier on those seeking entry into the industry than on already established provider institutions. For example, controls on expansion of acute care beds seldom distinguish between beds operated by a conventional short term hospital and those owned by or dedicated for use by an HMO. As a result, if conventional providers have saturated the market with beds, regulation of beds will block HMO development, whereas straight unregulated competition might permit the HMO to crowd out other, more costly forms of care.

Second, advocates of HMOs and other innovations argue that health planners and regulators are persuaded and coerced by existing providers to discriminate against new entries that will "harm" the existing health care system, even though such innovations promise higher quality, lower cost care. The data presented in Chapter two do not support this contention, but perhaps only because few innovations have reached the stage of formal proposals.

The vision of the future embodied in PL 93-641 and most state health plans and regulatory programs is that of a health care system that is less dependent on expensive inpatient care and that emphasizes preventive medicine. However, the simple truth is that neither the federal legislation nor state programs actually contain money or authority to implement this vision.

State and Area Capacity

In the area of state and local capacity, the research presented in Chapter two tells an old, oft-repeated story of underinvestment in a public program resulting in performance so far below expectations that the very concepts underlying the program are brought into question. PL 93-641 compounds this problem by greatly expanding the mission of state and area health planning and regulatory agencies while, in the near term at least, actually reducing the resources available to many of these agencies. The handful of states that have pioneered a professional, reasonably sophisticated approach to regulation of the health industry—New York, Connecticut, Rhode Island, Maryland, Kentucky, and one or two others—all spend substantially more on staff and other resources than the federal funds made available to any state under PL 93-641.

The annual rate of investment in construction by nongovernment hospitals, based on unpublished building permit data assembled by the Bureau of Census, exceeds $1.5 billion. If investment by other types of providers, and equipment purchases and other forms of capital investment by hospitals were measured, total capital investment by institutional health care providers would surely exceed $2 billion annually. Yet, to regulate this enormous and, in terms of the public welfare, very crucial investment activity and to carry out comprehensive health planning functions, Congress authorized only $30 million for FY 1976—roughly 1.5% of the value of the investment to be reviewed. Federal financing appears even more inadequate if compared to total health care expenditures; the funds authorized by PL 93-641 for health planning and regulation in FY 1976 amount to only 1% of the *increase* in total health expenditures expected in 1977 alone.

The message of these figures seems clear—if there is sufficient public interest in controlling health capital investment and service development through universal CON regulation, that interest demands the appropriation of sufficient public funds to insure that regulation is competently administered. If CON regulation is at all effective as a cost containment device, it will easily save far more than $30 million each year in federal health costs alone, which now approach $30 billion annually.

Chapter 4

Legal Aspects of Health Facilities Regulation

Leonard H. Glantz

FEDERAL HEALTH PLANNING BACKGROUND

Public Law 93-641 is Congress's most recent attempt to regulate the health delivery system in the United States. Its enactment was based on Congress's perception of a number of forces that cause health care to be unevenly, unfairly, and inefficiently distributed to the public. Congress specifically found that the "highly technical nature of medical services together with the growth of third party reimbursement mechanisms act to attenuate the usual forces influencing the behavior of consumers with respect to personal health services."[1] In Chapter one, it was noted that since physicians decide which services the patient utilizes and third parties pay for such services, the patient's incentive to contain expenditure is reduced.

Additionally, Congress found that investments in costly health care resources are made without regard to the existence of similar facilities or equipment already in use in that area.[2] This practice has resulted in costly capital accumulation and the need to pay for underutilized services and equipment. While some areas offer expensive though underutilized services, other areas, such as inner cities and rural communities have an undersupply of needed medical services.[3]

Earlier chapters have touched on previous attempts to deal with this issue at the federal level. The most serious federal effort at cost containment prior to the enactment of PL 93-641 was the passage of the Section 1122 amendments to the Social Security Act in 1972.[4] Section 1122 provides that the Medicare, Medicaid, and maternal and child health programs will not support the construction of medical facilities unless the need for such facilities is established by a designated state planning agency. Unless need for a facility is established, these programs will not reimburse a facility for depreciation, interest, or return on equity capital relating to such unneeded capital expenditures.[5] Although Section 1122 does not prevent the construction of an unneeded facility, its requirement of the determination of need for a new facility has caused some to refer to it as the federal certificate of need law.

STATE CERTIFICATION OF NEED LAWS

The adoption of Section 1122 may to some extent demonstrate Congress's approval of the state CON laws. By the end of 1972 twenty states had adopted such statutes.[6] All these laws require that an administrative decision must be made that a need exists for a new facility or service prior to the construction of such facility or implementation of such service. The underlying philosophy is that such a prior determination of need will prevent duplication of services and the building of facilities that will not be used but must be paid for, and will ultimately lead to a more equitable distribution of health facilities and services.[7] In effect, CON laws are designed to correct perceived failures in the unregulated health services marketplace. In terms of economic theory and social policy, CON laws have been the subject of much criticism.[8] It is not the purpose of this chapter to comment on the validity of CON as a regulatory device. Whether or not CON programs are a wise idea, PL 93-641 requires states to adopt such programs if they wish to be eligible to receive certain federal funds in the future. Any state that has not entered into an agreement with the Secretary of HEW for the designation of a state agency by the end of the fourth fiscal year after the enactment of PL 93-641 may not receive any allotment, grant, loan, or loan guarantee under the Public Health Service Act, the Community Mental Health Center Act, or the Comprehensive Alcohol Abuse and Alcoholism Prevention, Treatment and Rehabilitation Act of 1970 for the development, expansion, or support of health resources in that state.[9] A designated state agency must administer a CON program[10] which has been adopted by the state.[11] Thus, in a relatively short period of time the majority of states will have to adopt a new system of health facilities regulation which they either did not consider adopting in the past, or did consider but rejected. One can expect a fair amount of litigation to arise out of this situation. It is our task to attempt to determine what type of legal challenges may develop, using past legal challenges as our guide.

THE CONSTITUTIONALITY OF CERTIFICATION OF NEED LAWS

The Police Power

As might be expected, the earliest constitutional attack on a certificate of need law occurred in New York, the first state to adopt such legislation. This law,[12] known as the Metcalf-McCloskey Act, established a State Hospital Review and Planning Council located with the Department of Health which, along with local hospital review and planning councils, made recommendations to the State Board of Social Welfare concerning the need for the construction of new nursing homes and hospitals. The establishment of a private proprietary nursing home could not be approved until the "public" need for such a home was established. The petitioners in the suit entitled *Attoma v. State Department of Social Welfare* [13] desired to open a nursing home, but for a number of complicated reasons did not receive approval to do so under the CON law. Upon appeal to the courts, it was alleged that the CON law was unconstitutional on the ground that the requirement that one must establish need for such a facility prior to receiving approval was not a reasonable exercise of the state's police power.[14] The "police power" is the power of the state to protect the health, safety, and welfare of its citizens. The New York court had little trouble dealing with this issue. It first discussed the fact that this statute was passed as the result of an "exhaustive study" by the state legislature. This study found that the uncontrolled construction of unnecessary or substandard hospital and nursing home beds may be one of the causes of spiraling health care costs. The court refused to overturn the legislation on this ground as long as there could be discovered "any state of facts either known or which could reasonably be assumed to afford support for the legislative decision to act."[15] It went on to find that the operation of a nursing home bore a reasonable relation to the health, safety, and welfare of a community and was therefore subject to licensing and regulation. Additionally, the court held that the "proliferation of such homes beyond the need" of an area would also affect the welfare of the community and, therefore, regulation on the basis of need was valid.

The outcome of this case was not particularly surprising. The regulation of the health care industry has been compared to the regulation of public utilities. It has been stated that these entities are analogous because,

> The business of health care is deeply and intimately affected with a public interest, because hospitals and like institutions have the power of exploitation in some measure, even though it is not frequently exercised, and because such instrumentalities carry on what is in some respects a natural monopoly. And it has long been recognized as a matter of economics as well as law, when a necessity of life is provided by a monopoly or quasi-monopoly, effective regulation of that enterprise is required to protect the public interest.[16]

Prior to commencing the construction of major facilities, beginning or terminating certain services, or undertaking certain other activities, public utilities must receive a certificate of public convenience and necessity. Justice Brandeis has stated that

> the purpose of requiring the certificate of public convenience and necessity is to promote the public interest by preventing waste. Particularly in those businesses in which interest and depreciation charges on plants constitute a large element in the cost of production, experience has taught that the financial burdens incident to unnecessary duplication of facilities are likely to bring high rates and poor service.[17]

There is a long history of courts' upholding the regulation of industries for the protection of the public good, and the extension of such regulation to the health care industry could not be said to be legally unwarranted.

There is, however, one case in which a state CON law was struck down as an unconstitutional exercise of the state's police powers. Because of this case's possible significance, it will be set forth in some detail. In *In Re Certificate of Need for Aston Park Hospital, Inc.,*[18] Aston Park Hospital filed an application for a CON under the applicable North Carolina statute,[19] for the construction of a 200-bed hospital in the city of Asheville. At the time of filing the application, the hospital operated a 50-bed institution located on one acre of land. It intended to cease operating this facility and replace it with a larger and more modern hospital to be located on a 69-acre tract which it owned at the time it filed the application. The state commission charged with determining need for new hospital facilities found that the insertion of a new 200-bed hospital into the Asheville area would produce "an unnecessary and weakening duplication of services and undesirable dilution of physicians' time in treating patients at widely separated hospitals."[20]

After spending a fair amount of time pointing out what this case did not involve, the court succinctly presented the issue as it perceived it.

> [Can a state constitutionally] forbid the construction, with private funds and suitable materials, upon private property suitably located, of a well planned hospital which is to be adequately equipped and staffed with a sufficient number of well trained personnel in all categories, the sole reason for such prohibition being that, in the opinion of the Commission, there are now in the area hospitals with bed capacity sufficient to meet the needs of the population[?][21]

The court found it could not.

The state argued that overbedding spreads the available limited supply of physicians, nurses, and other trained personnel too thinly, endangering the quality of patient care. Furthermore, it was alleged by the state that excess bed capacity increases the number of vacant rooms and beds, which tends to drive up the costs of care to patients in the occupied beds.

While acknowledging that the New York court found a similar argument persuasive in the *Attoma* case, the North Carolina court did not find it convincing. Instead it found, without citation to any authority, that:

> it is a matter of common knowledge that in many communities hospital costs have spiralled upward in recent years while patients desiring hospitalization have been unable to find promptly a vacant hospital room.[22]

By finding that compulsory curtailment of facilities for care of the sick is not a "reasonable choice of remedy" for a shortage of trained hospital personnel, the court revitalized the virtually totally discredited doctrine of "substantive due process." This doctrine had been used by the Supreme Court at the turn of the century to strike down economic regulation with which it disagreed.[23] In effect, the utilization of the substantive due process doctrine would enable a court to substitute its judgement for that of the legislature. The Court since that time has deferred to the Congress and has upheld such regulation as long as any state of facts could be conceived which would justify Congress's action. The North Carolina court, however, had no trouble substituting its judgement for that of the legislature's.

Specifically, the court found that forbidding a person to use his own funds and property to construct adequate facilities and employ a competent staff "merely because to do so endangers the ability of other, established hospitals to keep all their beds occupied"[25] violated Article I, § 19 of the North Carolina constitution, that constitution's due process clause.[26] To support this finding, the court continued to second-guess the legislature by observing that it has been the "common experience in America" that competition leads to lower prices, better service, and more efficient management, and that in this regard there is no reason to believe that hospitals are any different from other businesses.

The court recognized that utilities were regulated in a similar manner by the use of certificates of public convenience and necessity. However, it went on to point out that public utilities have their rates regulated in order to protect the public from the consequences of monopolies, and that hospital rates were not regulated.

Finally, the court found that the CON statute also offended Articles 32 and 34 of the North Carolina constitution which forbids the grant of exclusive privileges by the state and the establishment of monopolies.

Although a number of commentators were shocked by the action of the North Carolina court,[27] its impact should be of limited scope. First, the ruling held that the state CON law was contrary to the North Carolina constitution, not the United States Constitution. Second, the North Carolina court has a greater tendency than other courts to review policy decisions made by the state legislature.[28] This is especially true in economic regulation and occupational licensing cases.[29] Finally, this case is limited to the situation in which no public funds of any type are to be used for the construction of the hospital.

One aspect of this case is particularly confusing. At one point the court implies that the use of certificates of public convenience and necessity is a valid method of controlling public utilities, which it admits are monopolies, because the state also controls the rates these utilities charge.[30] This has led one commentator to state that if North Carolina regulated hospital rates, a CON law would be valid.[31] However, another analysis of the case concludes that even with rate regulation, the North Carolina court would strike down such laws.[32] In light of the constitutional analysis presented by the court, it would appear that the latter view would prevail.

One of the direct results of *Aston Park* is an attack by the state of North Carolina on the constitutionality of PL 93-641. In *North Carolina v. Mathews*[33] the state alleges, among other things, that PL 93-641 requires states to adopt a CON law or be penalized by losing substantial federal assistance, which will endanger the health of the people of North Carolina. It is further alleged that in order to comply with PL 93-641, it would have to amend its constitution since CON laws have been found unconstitutional in North Carolina by its supreme court, and that this places the legislative and constitutional processes of the state in the control of the United States Congress. The state argues that this violates Article IV, Section 4 (the guaranty clause) and the Tenth Amendment of the United States Constitution and the principles of federalism embraced in the Constitution.

At this point, no court has followed the *Aston Park* decision. The New Jersey court, in *Merry Heart Nursing and Convalescent Home v. Dougherty*[34] specifically rejected the holding in *Aston Park* stating, "we find the holding of that court not persuasive and at variance with the law of this State."[35] Furthermore, the court found that the power of a state to legislate in the field of public health is "no longer open to question" and, more specifically, that the CON requirement is a valid exercise of police power.[36]

Unconstitutional Delegation of Power

A standard method used to attack administrative decisions is to allege that the legislature's delegation of power to the administrative agency was unconstitutional. Congressional delegation of power to federal administrative agencies is virtually unassailable today. In only two cases, both decided in 1935, has the Supreme Court found a congressional delegation to be invalid.[37] As a leading authority on administrative law has stated,

> No responsible delegation is likely to be held unconstitutional. The non-delegation doctrine does not prevent delegation of legislative power. It does not prevent delegation of power to make law and to exercise discretion in individual cases. And it does not even assure meaningful legislative standards.[38]

The issue of the validity of a state legislature's authority to delegate its power to a state administrative agency is much less clear.[39] For the most part, state courts that have ruled on the issue based their determinations on the validity of the delegation of authority on whether or not the legislature has set forth adequate standards to control the scope of power of the administrative agency.[40] Modern courts are moving away from the legislative standards requirement, which has not proved to be either very useful or effective. Instead, the more modern courts are determining whether or not the administrative agency itself is providing individuals with adequate safeguards to assure that they are not subject to arbitrary and uncontrolled decisionmaking.[41]

There are two cases that deal with the problem of delegation in the context of CON legislation. In the New Jersey case previously discussed[42] the plaintiff alleged that the legislature gave the commissioner of public health unbridled discretion to establish his own standards, thereby abdicating its constitutional duty to establish standards. The court found that the statute established five general criteria for the issuance of certificates of need. They were:

(1) the availability of other facilities or services which may serve as alternatives or substitutes;

(2) the need for special equipment and services in the geographical area;

(3) the possible economies and improvements which could result from the operation of joint central services;

(4) the adequacy of financial resources of the applicant; and

(5) the availability of sufficient manpower in the several professional disciplines.[43]

The existence of these criteria was more than enough to sustain the delegation of power in this instance.

In the more interesting case of *Simon v. Cameron,* [44] the plaintiff contended that the California legislature unconstitutionally delegated its power to local planning agencies, which were private corporations, and that the standards for recommendations on CON applications were unconstitutionally vague. The local planning agencies were established under California law to review individual proposals for the construction of new health care facilities and to "make decisions as to the need and desirability for the particular proposal." [45] Unfavorable decisions by these local agencies could be appealed to the state-wide Health Planning Council, which was a "quasi-public" body, [46] composed of individuals who were appointed by the governor, the chairman of the senate rules committee, and the speaker of the assembly. Since the capability for an appeal existed, the court found that the local planning agencies had only initial decisionmaking authority delegated to it, with the final authority reposing in a body "responsible to" government officials and elected representatives. Although not mentioned by the court, the difference between initial and final decisionmaking power was relatively theoretical in California. Of the first 234 applications acted upon by the local agencies, only 13 appeals were filed. [47]

The court was not at all concerned with the fact that the local agencies were private corporations. It pointed out in one place in its decision that such agencies are "similar to other administrative agencies in the state," [48] and in another place that "the voluntary planning agency with its close state connections should be characterized as a public agency." [49] But even if the local planning agency was merely a private entity, the court cites numerous cases of legislative delegation to private parties. For example, the court pointed out that a number of states will license doctors only if they graduated from a medical school licensed by the Council on Medical Education, a nongovernmental body. In another example the court cited a case that upheld the delegation of licensing power by the Securities and Exchange Commission to the National Association of Securities Dealers. [50]

In finding that the delegation was not without adequate standards, the court found that the words "community need and desirability" were adequate standards, and were not vague or overbroad. In addition, the legislature required certain information to be given by license applicants, such as the population to be served, the utilization of existing programs, and the anticipated demand for the proposed health care services, and that this information was obviously intended to be among the factors which the local agency must consider in its determination of community need.

Thus, the delegation of authority to private corporations, which will be the legal structure of most HSAs, provided no problem. Very broad standards also provided no problem.

Anyone who plans to attack future CON decisions based on the unconstitutionality of the delegation of power due to lack of standards will have a very hard time of it. PL 93-641 sets forth the minimal criteria which must be considered in making such decisions, such as the need that the population to be served has for such services, the availability of less costly or more effective methods of providing such services, the availability of manpower, management personnel, and funds for capital and operating needs, the costs and methods of proposed construction, and so forth.[51] The criteria set forth in the law are more specific than the guidelines in the two cases just discussed. Furthermore, it can be expected that these criteria will be further defined in federal regulations.[52]

Vagueness

If a statute is so vague as to define insufficiently what action is being proscribed, it may be struck down as unconstitutional.[53] There is one case in which this problem arose in the CON situation. In *People v. Dobbs Ferry Medical Pavillion, Inc.*,[54] the definition of the term "clinic" was called into question. Shortly after the legalization of abortions in New York, three doctors formed a "partnership" for the practice of obstetrics, gynecology, and general surgery. More than three-fourths of their large practice consisted of the performance of abortions, with most of the patients coming from other states.

Shortly after opening these premises, an official from the public health department inspected the offices, concluded that they constituted a "hospital facility" and asked the physicians to file an application for approval. Upon their refusal to file such an application, an action for an injunction prohibiting the operation of the "hospital facility" was brought by the state.

At the trial the physicians contended that their offices did not constitute a hospital, but rather were merely a suite of offices. They also contended that the statute and regulations were unconstitutionally vague. The trial court, disagreeing with the physicians' position, enjoined them from conducting further abortions in their facilities. The appellate division reversed the trial court.

The New York public health law provided that no hospital could be established without the approval of the public health council and defined a hospital as:

> a facility or institution engaged principally in providing services by or under the supervision of a physician . . . for the prevention, diagnosis or treatment of human disease, pain, injury, deformity or physical condition . . . .[55]

Pursuant to its powers, the public health council further defined various medical facilities. Among these was the "independent out-of-hospital health facility" which was defined as:

> an institution with one or more health clinics not part of an inpatient hospital facility . . . which is primarily engaged in providing services and facilities to out-of-hospital or ambulatory patients by or under the supervision of a physician.[56]

The state claimed that the doctors' offices in question were actually an independent, out-of-hospital health facility. The dispute settled around the meaning of the term "clinic" as used in the definition of independent, out-of-hospital health facility.

The court started its analysis by setting forth the law regarding vagueness as stated by the United States Supreme Court—a law "forbidding or requiring conduct in terms so vague that men of common intelligence must necessarily guess at its meaning and differ as to its application violates due process of law."[57] With this rule of law as its guide, the court went on to analyze the facts in the case.

None of the state's witnesses attempted to define the term "clinic," and the state apparently assumed that everyone, especially doctors, knew what it meant. Neither Stedman's Medical Dictionary nor Webster's Dictionary provided any guidance, in that their definitions could include hospitals or private doctors' offices. Defense witnesses argued that the term was practically indefinable and very loosely used. For example, they testified, both the Mayo Clinic and Leahy Clinic were, in fact, group practices.

Thus, it appeared to the court that the term "clinic" and "group practice" were virtually interchangeable. Since private group practices were not subject to hospital regulation in New York, the state could not convert a group practice into a "hospital" merely by calling it a clinic. Since the term "clinic" was so vague, the court determined that the law and regulations taken together were unconstitutional as written and applied in this case.

The dissenting judge argued that physicians do know what the term "clinic" means and that the law, therefore, was not vague. He argued that when someone went to a *place* for treatment instead of to a doctor, that one would be dealing with an institution. The fact that so many of the patients of this practice came from out of state indicated to this judge that they were going to a place, and not a doctor, for treatment, and that this would make it a clinic.[58]

The New York Court of Appeals affirmed the ruling that the statute and regulations were unconstitutionally vague.[59] More specifically, they found that the statute and regulations were too broad in that the terms "facility" and "clinic" included a number of individual, partnership, and group practices that were not meant to be the subject of licensing. With proper draftmanship, however, such laws and regulations could be sustained.

PL 93-641 requires states to adopt CON programs that apply to "new institutional health services proposed to be offered or developed."[60] As we can see from the *Dobbs Ferry* case, such language might be fatally vague. As a result, HEW has proposed extensive regulations which greatly clarify this phrase. Thus the terms "to develop," "health care facility," "health services," "institutional health services," and "to offer" are all defined in considerable detail.[61] It is interesting to note, however, that even with such detailed regulations ambiguities will arise. For example, the regulations specifically state that "ambulatory surgical facilities" are to come under the jurisdiction of CON laws. They are defined as:

> a facility, not a part of a hospital, which provides surgical treatment to patients not requiring hospitalization. Such term does not include the offices of private physicians or dentists whether for individual or group practice.[62]

Assuming for the moment that abortion is a "surgical treatment," this definition could not help resolve the *Dobbs Ferry* case. The issue would still be whether or not these physicians were working in a "facility" or in their "offices." However, these regulations, which either explicitly or by implication will become part of every state's CON program, will be of great help in avoiding the "void for vagueness" problem.

An unusual bent to the problem of vagueness or overbreadth of a CON statute or regulation arises when an entity wishes to come under the mandate of the statute or regulation when it in fact does not. In many jurisdictions the state's Medicaid program establishes two rates, one for physicians' office visits, and one for clinic or hospital outpatient visits. The latter rate is considerably higher than the former rate. To obtain the clinic rate one would have to be licensed, which requires going through the CON process. Thus some practitioners may wish to use the certification process to turn their group practice into a clinic,[63] thereby using the vagueness of the statute to their own advantage.

DUE PROCESS

In the making of public decisions, the public decision-maker, whether judge or administrative agency, must act fairly, impartially and non-arbitrarily. "Due process" encompasses all the requirements that are necessary to assure that decisions are made in a proper manner. These requirements are flexible, however, and may change depending on the circumstances and the type of decision to be made. For the purposes of this discussion, an agency administering a CON statute would be interested in obtaining two types of facts—adjudicative facts and legislative facts. An adjudicative fact is one about a party and his activities, business, and property. They usually answer the questions, who did what, when, where, how, and why. Legislative facts, on the other hand, usually do not concern the immediate parties but are generally facts that help the decision-maker decide questions of law and policy.[64] One of the very basic due process rights is a person's right to a hearing on an issue that affects that person. The question is, however, to what kind of hearing is that person entitled?

Generally there are two types of hearings—a "trial-type" hearing and an "argument-type" hearing. The trial-type hearing is usually required when one attempts to make a finding of adjudicative fact. Thus, evidence is presented by witnesses, and the witnesses are confronted and cross-examined. In this situation the facts usually concern an individual, and the individual should be able to present his own evidence and confront those who present negative evidence.[65]

In determining legislative facts a trial-type hearing is usually not required. In such a situation the agency is merely trying to ascertain information it needs to make broad policy decisions that affect a number of people. In this sense the agency will be acting like a legislature prior to passing a law.

Legislative fact finding is amply demonstrated in a case in which the Civil Aeronautics Board adopted a rule stating that only all-cargo airlines could sell cargo space at wholesale rates under certain circumstances.[66] A passenger airline that was dissatisfied with this ruling argued that a trial-type hearing was required prior to the adoption of such a rule. The court pointed out that the CAB had received written materials and had heard arguments prior to adopting the rule, and that the petitioners could not explain what types of facts would be brought out in a trial-type hearing. The determination of the question at issue did not depend on the characteristics of the party that was unhappy with the CAB's decision, but rather on the economic situation of the industry in general.

In contrast, the case of *Willner v. Committee on Character*[67] is a pure example of adjudicative fact finding that required a trial-type hearing. *Willner* concerned the case of a person who passed the New York bar examination, but who was refused admission to the bar because of the Committee on Character's finding that he did not possess the character and personal fitness to be an attorney. This finding was made without giving the applicant an opportunity for a hearing prior to such a denial, or any chance for the applicant to show why such a denial was unwarranted. The determination in this case was made on the basis of findings about the character of the applicant, about his past activities and present trustworthiness. Thus, the Supreme Court found that he should have been given an opportunity to be heard and to confront witnesses.[68]

Both PL 93-641[69] and the proposed regulations[70] require a "public hearing" in the course of state agency or HSA review of a CON application if requested by a person directly affected by the review. No guidance is given as to whether this requires a trial-type hearing or an argument-type hearing. In order to resolve this problem one must determine whether legislative or adjudicative facts are required prior to the issuance or denial of a CON. There is probably no question that one must always make a determination of legislative facts prior to this situation. Indeed, this is partially done through the adoption of the Health Systems Plan (HSP) and the Annual Implementation Plan (AIP).[71] In addition to this information, however, the agency might need to ascertain more detailed information concerning the health needs in the applicant's area and the existing resources. This still looks like legislative fact finding. Thus, if a state agency denies an applicant's request for the construction of 25 surgical beds on the grounds that such beds are not needed because of the limited demands for such services, or because an overabundance of surgical beds in the applicant's service area presently exists, the denial would be based on legislative facts, and a trial-type hearing would not be required.

If, on the other hand, a hospital were denied the beds because it would not be capable of rendering adequate care, or because its funds are so mismanaged that the certifying agency does not believe its activities should be expanded, one would be dealing with adjudicative facts, and a trial-type hearing would be required if requested by the applicant.

In *Milligan v. Board of Registration in Pharmacy*[72] two individuals were denied a permit to open a drug store. Under the applicable statute[73] such a permit could only be denied if the board found that such a store would be inconsistent with the best interests of the public health, welfare, or safety. The court noted that the effect of the denial was to preclude qualified pharmacists from pursuing a lawful vocation at places where they deemed it advantageous to work. In order for the board to deny such a permit, it would have been required to make a determination of "facts concerning each applicant and the place in which he wishes to carry on business."[74] In such a case a trial-type hearing would be necessary. The questions involved were predominantly adjudicative—"the objective ascertainment of facts about the applicants, their capacity, their reliability, their ability to conduct and finance a drug store, suitability of the premises, and like matters."[75]

It can be said with some certainty that when a CON decision is based on facts unique to the applicant, a trial-type hearing may be required. This statement is supported by a decision of the Massachusetts Health Facilities Appeals Board, the administrative appeals body for CON decisions, in which it was found that when a denial of a CON was based on the applicant's past performance, moral character, and prior revocation of a license, a trial-type hearing was required.[76] Such a finding is not a determination of need, in the strict sense of the term. It could be found that a hospital or nursing home is needed in the area, but that the applicant is not personally qualified to operate such an institution. Such a finding requires a trial-type hearing.

Another requirement of due process is that the decision-maker arrive at his decision on the basis of ascertainable standards. This reduces the possibility of abuse of discretionary power, reduces arbitrariness, and informs applicants of what they must do or prove to be successful in their application.[77] A good example of this requirement is found in *Holmes v. N.Y. City Housing Authority*.[78] This case was brought by individuals who had applied for admission to public housing but had their application rejected. It was shown that the housing authority annually received 90,000 applications for 10,000 vacant apartments. However, the authority had adopted no standards for the selection process. The court found that the absence of standards leads to the existence of absolute and uncontrolled discretion, which constituted an intolerable invitation for abuse.[79] Due process required the setting of some standards, even if it consisted only of drawing lots or admitting people on a chronological basis.

The problem of standards is addressed by PL 93-641 and the proposed regulations which require that all HSA and state agency reviews be conducted in accordance with certain criteria.[80] Indeed, the proposed federal regulations *require* a state to make certain findings prior to granting the issuance of a CON for inpatient facilities. Among these required findings are,

a) that less costly, more efficient or more appropriate alternatives to such inpatient service are not available and the development of such alternatives has been studied and found not practicable . . .;

c) that in the case of new construction, alternatives to new construction (e.g., modernization or sharing arrangements) had been considered . . .;

d) that patients will experience serious problems in obtaining inpatient care of the type proposed in the absence of the proposed new service. . . .[81]

The good faith utilization of such specific criteria will assure that all applicants will be treated fairly and equally.

The statute requires that in the review of all applications, the HSA and state agency first establish the relationship of the health services being reviewed to the applicable HSP and AIP. The adoption of the HSP is probably the most important planning activity performed by the HSA. The HSP is a detailed statement of goals describing a healthful environment in the health systems area which, when developed, will assure that quality health services will be available to all residents of the area at a reasonable cost. The HSP must be responsive to the unique needs and resources of the area and must be consistent with national health planning policy.[82] There is also a formal HSP adoption procedure set out in the act. A public hearing must be held, and all persons must be given an opportunity to present their views orally and in writing. This is a pure case of finding legislative facts and would not be a trial-type hearing. Upon adoption of the HSP there would be a definable set of standards against which applications could be reviewed.

The question has arisen as to whether or not the reviewing agency is absolutely tied to a plan it uses in reviewing CON applications. In the *Merry Heart* case discussed earlier,[83] New Jersey had adopted a state plan regarding the number of nursing home beds that New Jersey required. On March 9, 1972 the plan was published in the New Jersey *Register* which stated that there was a need for 336 additional nursing home beds in the applicant's area. This plan was based on data compiled through March 31, 1971. On March 21, 1972 the plaintiff submitted his application to the New Jersey Department of Public Health. On June 2, 1972 the plan was updated, at which time it was stated that 460 nursing home beds had been added to the applicant's region, resulting in an excess number of beds, and eliminating the need for additional facilities. On August 15, 1972 the applicant was notified that his application was denied because there was no need for additional beds at that time. The applicant was given a hearing on this rejection. The applicant alleged, and the hearing officer found, that the application should be reviewed on the basis of the March 9, 1972 published plan and not on the plan that was updated after the application was filed. This finding was appealed by the Department of Public Health.

The applicant's basic contention was that the use of the updated statistics would deprive it of due process of law. The court found that there was no question but that for an agency rule (which includes a health plan) to be effective it must be published and filed with the secretary of the state as required by New Jersey law.[84] This was not done for the June 1972 update of the plan. The issue before the court, then, was whether the change in the plan to reflect current statistical data was such an amendment as to require formal amendment procedures before such data could be utilized. The court found it was not.[85]

The statute required the adoption of a health plan to carry out the policy of the state that hospital and related services of "the highest quality, of a demonstrated need efficiently provided and properly utilized at a reasonable cost are of vital concern to the public health."[86] To do this the commissioner of public health was directed to conduct surveys and studies concerning the need for health care facilities and to "keep current records and statistics thereon."[87] The purpose of the plan was to determine the needs in each area for different types of facilities. There was no question that the building of new facilities or the closing of old facilities affected the needs of the regions and therefore the statistics were subject to change. The court found that the mere change in such statistics did not require formal adoption of amendments to the plan.

The use of updated data did not impinge on the applicant's due process rights. It was available at all times to the applicant. In addition, the applicant could contest the reliability of the department's information at its hearing by cross-examining witnesses and introducing its own evidence on the needs of the region. The determination by the commissioner would then be made on all available evidence.

This case would seem to imply that the HSP will not handcuff the agencies reviewing applications for CON since updated data could be used. However, more serious changes in the review criteria without adequate procedures could lead to problems. In the *Dobbs Ferry* case, wherein it was determined that the term "clinic" was unconstitutionally vague, the court ruled that the problem with the statute was "compounded by the fact that, as applied by the State Health Department, the sweep of the statute and code is determined by the changeable, unpublished directives of the changeable administration of the Health Department."[88]

WRITTEN FINDINGS, REASONS, AND
SUBSTANTIAL EVIDENCE

PL 93-641 requires that all HSA and state agencies adopt procedures for making "written findings which state the basis for any final decision or recommendation made by the agency or State agency."[89] This requirement greatly reduces the opportunity for arbitrary action by forcing the agency to explain the basis for its action.[90] Although the Supreme Court originally based its requirement of written finding on the Constitution, this is no longer the case.[91] There is a strong practical reason for requiring written findings, however—it greatly simplifies judicial review. Unless an agency specifically pinpoints the grounds upon which it made its decision, a court would have to go through the entire and often voluminous record to determine if the decision is sound. It also keeps the courts from becoming fact-finders, a task that is given to the agencies. Additionally, written findings help the parties plan their cases for rehearsing or judicial review.[92]

Once an agency has made its findings, applied the standards it must use, and made its decision, agency action is usually subject to judicial review. Assuming there are no allegations of procedural irregularities, the appellant will usually argue that the decision reached was not based on substantial evidence.[93] Substantial evidence means "such relevant evidence as a reasonable mind might accept as adequate to support a conclusion."[94] It is really a determination of whether or not the administrative agency acted reasonably in light of all the facts. Even if a court disagrees with the decision of the agency, it should not reverse it if the agency acted reasonably.

A determination of substantial evidence will not only take into account the amount of evidence, but the type of evidence. Thus, "mere uncorroborated hearsay or rumor does not constitute substantial evidence."[95] There are times when a court will review the substantive basis of a decision under the guise of determining if the evidence was adequately substantial to uphold an agency decision. In *Schware v. Board of Bar Examiners*[96] an individual was not admitted to the bar because of a finding that he was unfit to practice law. The bar examiners found that the applicant was a communist, had used aliases, and had a history of arrests. The Court found that "there is no evidence in the record which rationally justifies a finding that Schware was morally unfit to practice law."[97] The Court did not find that the evidence was insufficient to prove that Schware was arrested or used aliases, but that these incidents should not be grounds for exclusion from the bar. It was really critical of the standards utilized, and not the findings that were made. This point was made in Justice Frankfurter's concurring opinion.[98]

The requirement for written findings by the state agency is important not only for applicants, but also for the HSA which has made recommendations to the state agency. If a state agency decides to issue a CON to a facility, which decision is not consistent with the HSP or AIP of the HSA, the state agency must submit to the HSA a detailed statement of the reasons for this inconsistency.[99] The HSA may then appeal that decision under an appeals mechanism consistent with state law.[100] In the absence of a written detailed statement of the reasons for the inconsistency, such a right to appeal would be severely abridged.

It is interesting to note that the HSA's right to appeal is an expansion of a traditional rule of standing. Generally, only an aggrieved party may file an appeal. The question has arisen as to whether or not an administrative agency that makes CON decisions has such standing. In a Minnesota case[101] the state Board of Health refused to issue a CON and the appeals board reversed the decision and ordered a certificate to be issued. The Board of Health appealed to the courts under a statute giving "any aggrieved person" the right to appeal.[102] The court found that an agency that functions in a judicial or quasi-judicial capacity is without the right to appeal, since it is in no different position than a court or a judge which has rendered a decision. No hard and fast rule was set down as to when an agency would be deemed to be functioning in a judicial or quais-judicial capacity. The court did say that when the function under consideration involved the exercise of discretion and required notice and hearing, the agency would be acting in a quasi-judicial fashion.[103] It was also said that an agency acts in a quasi-judicial fashion when it applies law to facts or when it resolves controversies between other entities of government or individual members of the public. Whether an agency could act on its own or had to wait for parties to appeal before it could act, was also deemed to be significant.[104] Under these tests it is highly probable that an HSA would not have standing to appeal a state agency's decision. The act specifically gives it this right, which is made all the more enforceable by requiring written findings and reasons of the state agency.

COMPETING APPLICATIONS

The situation will almost certainly arise when two facilities hope to be issued a CON to provide similar services. This does not mean that two applications have been filed simultaneously, but that the agency is aware of the fact that in addition to the applicant, there is another facility that intends to file an application for a CON. Although not discussed in the law, this problem is implicitly addressed in the proposed regulations. It is provided that in the course of agency review, a "person directly affected" by the services may request a public hearing.[105] Included in the definition of the term "person directly affected" is a health care facility that has "formally indicated an intention to provide such similar services in the future, either through the filing of a letter of intent or by adoption of a plan."[106] Thus, a person who has formally demonstrated an intention to provide services similar to those proposed by the applicant has a right to ask for a hearing. The question of what type of hearing again arises.

A similar situation was found in the case of *Delta Airlines, Inc. v. Civil Aeronautics Board*.[107] The applicable statute required a hearing on an application by an airline that desired to operate a new route. There were applications pending that would have covered the same route as the one under consideration. The airlines contended that if an affirmative decision were reached on one application prior to their receiving a hearing, the hearing would be meaningless when held. Or to put it another way, if A airline and B airline apply to operate the same route, and A's application is granted prior to B's hearing, and only one airline can operate on that route, then, in effect, B's application has been denied without B's having a hearing. The court found that A's application could not be granted without giving B a hearing. This finding follows the Supreme Court's "Ashbacker Doctrine" which held that when the Federal Communications Commission had two mutually exclusive applications pending, the FCC could not grant one without granting a hearing to the other.[108]

Under the proposed regulations, it appears that if X hospital has applied for a CON and Y hospital has previously filed a letter communicating its intention to provide a similar service, then Y can request a hearing on X's application. Assuming that it has already been determined that 25 new surgical beds are needed in the area and either X or Y could provide these beds, the only issue would be which one is better able to provide the services. This would require a finding of adjudicative facts, and a trial-type hearing would then be required. This type of proceeding would tend to get rather complicated, but it would be especially important here to protect the rights of both parties. To do this, some standards would have to be adopted so that the choice of one hospital over the other would not be arbitrary.[109]

ADMINISTRATIVE AND POLITICAL OVERREACHING

It is a basic rule that administrative agencies can act only within the scope of their mandate from the legislature, and any action beyond that mandate is improper and invalid. As an obvious example, the Interstate Commerce Commission may not resolve labor-management disputes which are within the jurisdiction of the National Labor Relations Board. Of course, much subtler problems of this nature can arise, and have arisen in the CON context.

In Massachusetts the issue has arisen in the context of the Department of Public Health's placing conditions on the issuance of CON.[110] Sometimes, when this comes about as a result of informal discussion, no conflict arises between the applicant and the department. Thus, when Holyoke Hospital applied for a CON for 55 new hospital beds in an already overbedded region, the department and the hospital, through consultation with each other, scaled down the application. The hospital was permitted to convert 19 obstetrical beds into 13 medical/surgical beds and 6 coronary care beds. The 19-bed conversion was conditioned on the hospital's agreement to close down its underutilized maternity service and to work with other hospitals in the area to continue to provide high quality obstetrical and gynecological services.[111] Both the hospital and the Department of Public Health were satisfied with the outcome of this process.

This amicable outcome is in contrast to another case involving Somerville Hospital, which desired to renovate completely its antiquated facilities. Because the wooden frame structure of the building placed it in violation of state safety requirements, denial of the CON would have led to its closing. The "A" and "B" agencies recommended approval and suggested that Somerville enter into planning with nearby Central Hospital with the objective of better coordination of services. However, an independently commissioned study by the department recommended that Somerville buy Central and close it down. After lengthy legal proceedings, Somerville was finally granted its CON four years after its initial application.[112]

Strictly speaking, the department never actually "conditioned" Somerville's CON on the purchase and closing of Central, but it came as close to this as one possibly could. It is not at all clear that the department had the statutory power to set conditions on the issuance of a CON. The statute does not give the department the authority to close inefficient or underutilized hospitals or departments of hospitals. Yet, by setting conditions, it could do just that. Additionally, if an institution applies for ten new pediatric beds, and it is determined that such beds are needed in the hospital's service area, can the application for these be denied because the hospital has an underutilized maternity department?[113] Given proper legislative authority, there is no question that state agencies could place

conditions on the issuance of a CON. But this should be a legislative decision and not an administrative one.

Besides administrative abuses, political abuses are also bound to find
their way into the regulatory system.[114] A case of this sort has been decided in Massachusetts. The Bessie Burke Memorial Hospital in Lawrence, Massachusetts was denied a CON, and this denial became an issue
in that city's 1973 mayoral election. Community pressure continued to
rise, culminating in the introduction of special legislation by the Lawrence state representative. This legislation,[115] passed over the governor's
veto ordered the Department of Public Health to issue a CON notwithstanding the provisions of the CON statute.[116] The commissioner of
public health filed an action to overturn this legislation.[117] The commissioner alleged that the special enactment violated Article X and Article
XXX of the Massachusetts Declaration of Rights since it gives special
privileges to one individual and permits the legislature to exercise the
powers of the executive in violation of separation of powers. He also
argued that it violated the 14th Amendment of the United States Constitution. The court, however, upheld the constitutionality of the enactment. The court cited its own cases to demonstrate that Article X does
prohibit special treatment by the legislature. In *Holden v. James,* referring to Article X, it was stated:

> It is manifestly contrary to the first principle of civil liberty and
> natural justice, and to the spirit of our constitution and laws,
> that any one citizen should enjoy privileges and advantages,
> which are denied to all others under like circumstances; or that
> anyone should be subjected to losses, damages, suits or actions,
> from which all others under like circumstances are exempted.[118]

Similar statements cited were found in other cases.[119] However, the
court found that in those cases the granting of a special privilege to one
person would detrimentally affect another. In one case[120] the legislature
enacted a special law exempting an individual from the requirement that
special notice be given to a municipality as a condition of an action
against it for negligence. By waiving this requirement the muncipality
would suffer direct harm as it could now be sued, whereas prior to the
enactment it could not. In *Bessie Burke* the court found that if special
legislation aiding one party did not injure another, it would be valid. The
court recognized that an enactment permitting excessive or misguided
construction could cast needless expense on the members of the public
"who foot the bill in the long run." But this was not deemed to cause
specific harm to identifiable individuals and, therefore, did not offend
Article X. Thus, the court found that if special legislation injures one per-

son it is impermissible, but if it injures a large number of people it must be allowed to stand. It would appear that if one person in the city of Lawrence complained that such a law would cause him to receive insufficient care at a higher cost, or if one competitor showed that it would be denied expansion of its facilities in the future as a result of this special enactment, that it would then be unconstitutional.

The issue of whether the legislature can require the executive branch to take specific action was dealt with in much the same manner. The legislature can cause an action to be taken or supercede an administrative decision as long as it does not work an injury upon a private right. For example, in one case the Industrial Accident Board decided a controversy in favor of an insurance company and against an injured employee. The legislature passed special legislation ordering the commission to rehear the case. Since the legislation might have worked to the injury of the insurance company, it was found to be invalid. But the legislature can intervene in cases where it does not "interfere with distinct rights." By upholding such legislation, the court enabled the legislature to disrupt the regulatory and planning process and to demoralize those responsible for such regulation and planning.

Although PL 93-641 cannot prevent legislatures from acting in this manner, it can go a long way in dissuading them from passing such legislation. Under PL 93-641 the governor of a state must, as part of the designation agreement, assert that the state agency shall carry out the health planning and development functions as prescribed in §1523. Part of those functions is to administer the required state CON program. Under PL 93-641 the CON program must provide that the state agency must make a determination of need prior to health facility construction so that "only those services, facilities and organizations found to be needed shall be offered or developed in the State."[121] In the Bessie Burke case just discussed, the legislature required the issuance of a CON notwithstanding the fact that it was found by all the reviewing agencies that no need existed. Such an action could be taken as a breach of the designation agreement, which may be grounds for termination of the agreement by the secretary of HEW[122] or a refusal to renew the agreement[123] with the consequent loss of federal funds to that state.

PROBLEMS OF HSA GOVERNING BOARD COMPOSITION AND CONFLICT OF INTEREST

PL 93-641 delineates the composition of the HSA governing board. A majority, but not more than 60 percent, of the board must be residents who are consumers of health care and who broadly represent a number of constituencies.[124] One of the HSA's functions is to assist the state agency in fulfilling its CON function by reviewing and making recommendations respecting the need for new institutional health services proposed in its area.[125] In performing this task the HSA must hold hearings if requested, take testimony, give written notice to affected persons, and so on. One way it might be possible for an unsuccessful applicant to attack a decision of the state agency would be to allege that the HSA board that made a recommendation was improperly composed when the recommendation was made, that this recommendation was therefore invalid, and that the state agency should not have considered it in making its decision. One might also be able to attack the HSP upon which the recommendation was made by arguing that the board which adopted the HSP was improperly constituted.

The problem regarding board composition will probably be directed toward the consumer members. Although the term "consumer" is not defined in the act, the term "provider" is defined, and anyone who is not a provider is a consumer. The definition of provider includes any "indirect provider," which is the term that will cause most of the mischief. For example, anyone who receives more than one-tenth his gross annual income, either directly or through his spouse from an "entity engaged in the provision of health care" is an indirect provider. The word "entity" produces a problem as it is a term of broad sweep. If a law professor works for a university that has a medical school or teaching hospital, is the "entity" providing health care the university or the medical school? If it is the university, then the law professor is an indirect provider, as is the football coach, janitorial staff, and anyone else who works for the university. The policeman who works for a city that owns and operates a city hospital may also be an indirect provider.

In terms of conflicts of interest, however, it is the provider members of the board who will run into problems. The federal regulations on health systems agencies require HSA bylaws to contain a provision relating to conflicts of interest which will preclude use of membership on the governing body for purposes which are, or give the appearance of being, motivated by private gain.[126] Conflict of interest or bias refers not to a point of view, but to a direct personal interest in the outcome of a proposal. Thus, judges who think murder is a reprehensible act are not prohibited from conducting a murder trial, but a judge who owns stock in a corporation whose fortunes will rise or fall depending on the outcome of a trial may not conduct that trial.[127] If an HSA board member has direct interest, either as a supporter or a competitor, in the outcome of a CON application, he should not participate in that decision. Such a bias might nullify the recommendation of the entire board.

It is proper to ask at this point, if the HSA merely makes recommendations, can't the recommendations be disregarded if improperly made, thereby negating any adverse consequences of the improperly made recommendations? It appears that the HSA does more than make mere recommendations. The HSA can appeal any decision of the state agency that is inconsistent with the HSA's recommendations.[128] That alone causes it to carry more weight than would a simple recommendation. Additionally, if the HSA has held a hearing on a CON application, the proposed federal regulations permit the state agency to waive its hearing.[129] This would make the HSA an important finder of facts, and the significance of its recommendation would be substantially increased.[130] If the state agency based its recommendations on these findings of fact, such a finding would have to be properly made by a properly constituted and unbiased body.

THE PROBLEM OF MINIMAL COMPLIANCE WITH THE LAW

Taken as a whole, the sections of PL 93-641 that deal with state agencies and HSAs set forth a complex decisionmaking process. The thrust of the act is to make the decisionmaking process as fair and as open to public scrutiny and participation as possible. The act, particularly Section 1532(b), and the proposed regulations describe the due process safeguards that have been discussed throughout this chapter.

The danger implicit in the act's specificity in this regard is that some will be tempted to follow the letter of the law but disregard its spirit. An example of this is the notice requirements found in the act. Prior to adopting an HSP the HSA must hold a hearing and publish a notice of such hearing in two newspapers of general circulation in the health service area.[131] The obvious intent of this section is to enable consumers and providers a chance to comment on the proposed HSP. As a result of this, a notice in the legal notices section of the newspapers may not suffice. It is common knowledge that the average person does not bother to read this section of the newspaper. It would therefore seem more appropriate to publish these notices in a section of the newspaper that is commonly read.

This same problem arises in the CON context. Both the law and regulations require that notification must be given to persons affected by the review of an application prior to conducting such review.[132] Notice to the public may be given by publication in newspapers of general circulation. The same problem of the reality of such notice arises in this context.

In one place in the regulations this problem is directly confronted. Prior to adopting review procedures and criteria, the state agency must publish a notice stating that such procedures are under consideration and request comments. The regulations specifically state that this notice "shall appear in other than the legal notices or classified advertisement sections of such newspapers."[133] The point to be made is that minimal and technical compliance with the due process provision of the act is going to cause problems for agencies and applicants, and will require the courts to resolve disputes that need not arise.

SUMMARY

Although CON laws have been with us for a relatively short period of time, a number of challenges have been made. While the specificity of PL 93-641 and its accompanying regulations will help avoid certain types of challenges in the future, it will cause others to arise. A large number of parties are involved, and different levels of responsibilities exist. The interrelations of these parties and the nature of their roles will undoubtedly be scrutinized, with final determinations being made by the courts.

Notes

1. S. REP. No. 93-1285, 93rd Cong., 1st Sess. and Ad. News 7842, 7878.
2. *Id.*
3. *Id.* at 7879.
4. P.L. 92-603, codified at 42 U.S.C. § 1320a-1.
5. 42 U.S.C. § 1320a-1(d)(1).
6. William Curran, "A National Survey and Analysis of State Certificate of Need Laws For Health Facilities," in *Regulating Health Care Facilities*, Clark Havinghurst, ed. (Washington, D.C.: American Enterprise Institute For Public Policy Research, 1974), p.85.
7. "The Certificate of Need Experience: An Early Assessment, Vol. 1: Summary Report" (Bureau of Health Services Research, Department of Health, Education and Welfare, 1974), p. 1.
8. *See, e.g.,* Clark Havighurst, "Regulation of Health Facilities and Services By 'Certificate of Need,'" *Virginia Law Review* 59 (1973): 1143; Richard Posner, "Certificate of Need For Health Care Facilities: A Dissenting View," in Havighurst, ed., *Regulating Health Care Facilities,* p. 113.
9. P.L. 93-641 § 1521(d).
10. P.L. 93-641 § 1523(a)(4)(B).
11. P.L. 93-641 § 1523(b)(2).
12. New York Laws, ch. 730 (1964).
13. 26 A.D.2d 12, 270 N.Y.S.2d 167 (1966).
14. *Id.* at 270 N.Y.S. 2d 171.

15. *Id.* at 171, citing Lincoln Building Assoc. v. Barr, 1 N.Y.2d 413, 415, 153 N.Y.S.2d 633, 635, 135 N.E.2d 801, 802.

16. A.J.G. Priest, "Possible Adaptation of Public Utility Concepts In The Health Care Field," *Law and Cont. Problems* 35 (1970): 839.

17. New State Ice Co. v. Liebman, 285 U.S. 262, 282 (1932) (Dissenting opinion) as cited in Priest, *id.* at 843.

18. 282 N.C. 542, 193 S.E.2d 729 (1973).

19. N. Car. Gen. St. Art. 21, ch. 90.

20. 193 S.E.2d at 730.

21. *Id.* at 733.

22. *Id.* at 734.

23. *See, e.g.,* Lochner v. New York, 198 U.S. 45 (1905).

24. *See, e.g.,* Nebbia v. New York, 291 U.S. 502 (1934).

25. 193 S.E.2d at 734.

26. Article I, § 19 reads:

> *Law of the land; equal protection of laws.* No person shall be taken, imprisoned, or disseized of his freehold, liberties, or privileges, or outlawed, or exiled, or in any manner deprived of his life, liberty, or property, but by the law of the land. No person shall be denied the equal protection of laws; nor shall any person be subjected to discrimination by the State because of race, color, religion, or national origin.

27. *See, e.g.,* William Curran, "A Severe Blow to Hospital Planning: 'Certificate of Need' Declared Unconstitutional," *New England Journal of Medicine* 288 (1973): 723.

28. Note, "Hospital Regulation After Aston Park: Substantive Due Process In North Carolina," 52 N.C. L. Rev. 772.

29. *Id.* at 772-779.

30. 193 S.E.2d at 734.

31. Curran, *supra* note 27.

32. Note, *supra* note 32 at 787.

33. No. 76-0049-Civ.-5 (E.D. N. Car., filed April 27, 1976).

34. 131 N.J. Super. 412 (1974).

35. *Id.* at 420.

36. *Id.* at 421.

37. Panama Refining Co. v. Ryan, 293 U.S. 388; A.L.A. Schecter Poultry Corp. v. United States, 295 U.S. 495.

38. Kenneth C. Davis, *Administrative Law Text* 27, 3rd ed. (St. Paul: West Publishing Co., 1972).

39. *Id.* at 36-41; Louis Jaffee, *Judicial Control of Administrative Action,* pp. 73-85 (Little, Brown and Co. Boston, 1965).

40. Davis, *supra* note 38 at 37-40.

41. *Id.* at 43.

42. Merry Heart *supra* note 34.

43. *Id.* at 424, citing N.J.S.A. 26:2H-8.

44. 337 F. Supp. 1380 (C.D. Cal. 1970).

45. Cal. Health and Safety Code § 437.7.

46. *Supra* note 44 at 1381.

47. "The Certificate of Need Experience Vol. II: State Reports, California" (Bureau of Health Services Research, Department of Health, Education and Welfare, 1974), p. 3.

48. *Supra* note 44 at 1381.

49. *Id.* at 1382.

50. *Id.* citing R.H. Johnson & Co. v. Securities Exchange Commission, 198 F.2d 690 (2d Cir. 1952).

51. P.L. 93-641 § 1532(c)(3)(4)(6)(9).

52. *See* 41 Fed. Reg. 11704 § 123.409 (March 19, 1976).

53. The "void for vagueness' doctrine is discussed in Antony Amsterdam, *The Void For Vagueness Doctrine in the Supreme Court,* 109 U. PA. L. REV. 67 (1960).

54. 40 A.D. 2d 324, 340 N.Y.S.2d 108 (1973).

55. *Id.* at 340 N.Y.S.2d 111, citing New York Public Health Law § 2801 (subd 1).

56. *Id.* citing § 700.2 of the New York Sanitary Code (10 C NYCRR 700.2).

57. *Id.* citing Baggett v. Bullitt, 377 U.S. 360, 367.

58. *Supra* note 54 at 340 N.Y.S.2d at 117.

59. People v. Dobbs Ferry Medical Pavillion, 33 N.Y.2d 584, 347 N.Y.S. 2d 452 (1973).

60. P.L. 93-641 § 1523(a)(4)(B).

61. 41 Fed. Reg. 11701-11702 § 123.401 (March 19, 1976).

62. Id. at § 123.401(b)(6).

63. See Robert Borsody, "State Certificate of Need Laws: Practical Problems of Compliance," *Journal of Legal Medicine* (Oct. 1975): 25.

64. This distinction was first offered in 1948 by Kenneth Culp Davis and is discussed in Davis, *supra* note 38 at 160.

65. *Id.* at 160-164.

66. American Airlines v. C.A.B., 359 F.2d 624 (1966).

67. 373 U.S. 96 (1963).

68. *Id.* at 102-103.

69. § 1532(a)(6).

70. 41 Fed. Reg. 11693 § 122.306(a)(7) and 11703 § 123.407(a)(7) (March 19, 1976).

71. P.L. 93-641 § 1513(b)(2)(3).

72. 348 Mass. 491, 204 N.E.2d 504 (1965).

73. Mass. Gen. Laws, Ch. 112 § 39.

74. *Supra* note 72 at 348 Mass. 499.

75. *Id.* at 501.

76. Milman v. Department of Public Health, Mass. Health Facilities Appeals Board 11, (June 14, 1973). And see, Bicknell v. Annas, Mass. Sup. Jud. Ct. No. 74-27 eq. (March 12, 1974).

77. See Davis, *supra* note 38 at 46-51.

78. 398 F.2d 262 (2d Cir. 1968).

79. *Id.* at 265.

80. § 1532(c).

81. 41 Fed. Reg. 11704 § 123.410 (March 19, 1976).

82. P.L. 93-641 § 1513(b)(2).

83. *Supra* note 34.

84. N.J.S.A. 52:14 B-2(e); N.J.S.A. 52:14 B-5.

85. *Supra* note 34 at 418.

86. *Id.*

87. *Id.*

88. *Supra* note 54 at 113.

89. § 1532(b)(6).

90. See Davis, *supra* note 38, p. 318.

91. *Id.* at 319.

92. *Id.* at 320-322.

93. *Id.* at 525 *et seq.*

94. Consolidated Edison Co. v. NLRB, 305 U.S. 197, 229 (1938).

95. *Id.* at 230.

96. 353 U.S. 232 (1956).

97. *Id.* at 247.

98. *Id.* at 249.

99. P.L. 93-641 § 1523(c).

100. P.L. 93-641 § 1522(b)(13).

101. Minnesota State Board of Health v. Governor's Certificate of Need Appeals Board, 230 N.W.2d 176 (Minn. 1975).

102. Minn. St. 15.0424, subd 1.

103. *Supra* note 101 at 179.

104. *Id.* at 179-180.

105. 41 Fed. Reg. 11703 § 123.407(a)(7).

106. *Id.* at § 123.407(a)(7)(1).

107. 275 F.2d 632 (D.C. Cir. 1959).

108. Ashbacker Radio Co. v. F.C.C. 326 U.S. 327 (1945).

109. *See* Holmes v. N.Y. City Housing Authority, *supra* note 78.

110. Alan Reider, John Mason and Leonard Glantz, "Certificate of Need: The Massachusetts Experience," *American Journal of Law and Medicine* 1 (1975): 21.

111. *Id.* pp. 22-23.

112. *Id.* at 25-28.

113. A good argument can be made that the cost of pediatric beds will be higher because they will be forced to subsidize the underutilized maternity beds and therefore such review is valid.

114. *See* Havighurst, *supra* note 8 at 1204.

115. St. 1973, ch. 923.

116. *See* Reider, *et al., supra* note 110 at 32 n.82.

117. Commissioner of Public Health v. The Bessie M. Burke Memorial Hospital, Mass. 1975 Adv. Sh. 253, 323 N.E.2d 309 (1975).

118. *Id.* at Adv. Sh. 264, citing 11 Mass. 396 (1815).

119. *Id.*

120. Paddock v. Brookline, 347 Mass 230 (1964).

121. § 1523(a)(4)(B).

122. § 1521(b)(2)(C).

123. § 1521(b)(4).

124. § 1512(b)(3)(C)(i).

125. § 1513(f).

126. 41 Fed. Reg. 12826 § 122.104(b)(1)(ix) (March 26, 1976).

127. *See* Davis, *supra* note 38, chap. 12.

128. § 1522(b)(13).

129. 41 Fed. Reg. 11703 § 123. 407(a)(7)(ii).

130. *See* Simon v. Cameron, *supra* note 44 at 1382 wherein local health planning agencies were described as fact-finders.

131. § 1513(b)(2)(C).

132. § 1532(b)(1); 41 Fed. Reg. 11703 § 123.407(a)(1).

133. 41 Fed. Reg. 11703 § 123.406(b)(2).

Chapter 5

Methods Used in Determining Health Service and Facility Requirements

Robert M. Crane

This chapter was written by Robert M. Crane in his private capacity. No official support or endorsement by the Health Resources Administration of HEW is intended or should be inferred.

INTRODUCTION

Central to carrying out the effective regulation of services and facilities as called for in the CON and Section 1122 processes is the ability to determine the types and amount of health care services that a population will require. The determination of the need and demand of a population for services is a basic part of any institution's long range plan and is likely to be reflected in the goals which it establishes. As such, statements about the need and demand for services would be prominent in any hospital's application for a CON. The designers of programs would logically respond to the evidence of present and future need and demand.

Similarly, a major part of a Health Systems Agency's (HSA) or State Health Planning and Development Agency's (SHPDA) work is the determination of the types of services that are required to provide a population with adequate medical care. This determination will be reflected in the HSA's Health Systems Plan and Annual Implementation Plan and the State Health Plan approved by the Statewide Health Coordinating Council. These plans will also make some estimate of the facility and other resources required to provide these services.

The basis for making the CON determination is likely also to be reflected in the criteria and standards adopted by the HSA or SHPDA for use in reviewing new institutional health services and conducting other review activities. The question of whether adequate services are available can be partially answered by applying one or some combination of the methods described below. Criteria are also likely to reflect accessibility, quality, acceptability, continuity, and cost questions. The answers to these will help the agency make judgements about where new services should be developed and by whom. Such criteria will be adopted in a public process so that interested parties can influence the agency's selection of these decisionmaking guides.

While each institution or agency will make some determination about the need and demand for services and facilities as part of its planning and the CON or 1122 process, the methods used to arrive at this determination can vary. An attempt will be made to describe several of the major need determination methodologies that are currently being used.[1]

NEED OR DEMAND

The first question to be answered in thinking about determining the need for health services and facilities is, what do we want to try to measure and project—need or demand? The words *need* and *demand* are used interchangeably by many, yet they have very specific and different meanings.

Need

Need refers to some level of health services that ought to be consumed during a period of time in order to attain a desired level of health status. Need can be professionally or individually defined. Ordinarily, need is determined by professional judgement, usually physician. As such, need can vary just as do practice patterns which reflect the absence of concensus concerning when and how best to treat illness. For example, different treatment modes—radiation therapy or chemotherapy—may be acceptable and effective in improving the health status of cancer patients. The choice of one as opposed to another may have a dramatic effect on the resources required—facilities, equipment and manpower.

On an individual level, a need occurs when a person's perceived health status is different enough from his expected health status that he begins to think about entering the health care system to seek treatment. This felt need is a result of various psychological, social, and cultural factors which interrelate and affect an individual's beliefs and attitudes about illness and the desire for health care.[2]

Need is very difficult to measure from both an individual and professional perspective. Ordinarily, a relationship is established between the sociodemographic characteristics of a population and the mortality and morbidity rates of that population. Data on the causes and rates of death or illness of a specific population are used to infer the health needs of similar populations. Estimates are then made of the health services and related resources that are required to provide for these services. Method E in the next section amplifies on this.

When used as a basis for predicting bed and service requirements from the medical standpoint, need will most likely result in an overestimation of potential utilization since not all need is, or can be, translated into demand. Need from an individual viewpoint is difficult to measure since it is defined differently by every individual and reflects the individual's perception of health and illness. As compared to professionally defined need, it could lead to both underutilization or misutilization of services.

Demand

When an individual perceives that he is ill—that his current health status is different from his expected health status—and he desires to improve his health status, he is described as having a felt need. If he decides to seek care and initiates contact with a health practitioner, he has entered the health care system and translated his felt need into effective demand.[3] Effective demand for health services is, thus, defined as that quantity of services actually used by an individual or group.

In economic terms, the demand function is the relationship between quantities of goods and services, prices, and incomes. The demand for health services is that quantity of services demanded for any given price, all other things (e.g., income and preferences) being equal. That quanity which is actually demanded (effective demand) is the amount of services purchased at a certain price during some specified period of time.[4] Such economic analysis as applied to health planning quickly becomes complicated for many reasons. For example, in an emergency, felt need is likely to be translated into demand regardless of price. People invariably pay for health services indirectly through insurance. Thus, price at the time of service is low or zero; and for many services the physician acts for the patient to demand services.[5] For planning purposes, however, effective demand, which here will be referred to simply as demand, is equated with and measured by utilization. Utilization is much easier to measure than the factors associated with need, and planners are primarily interested in planning for those needs that will be expressed. Thus, most methods that are in wide use are focused on demand.

Problems, however, are inherent in the simple measurement and projection of demand. Consideration must be given to those factors that can affect demand. For example, the availability and acceptability of substitutes such as long term care for acute inpatient care, a change in price or reduction of financial barriers (passage of national health insurance), inappropriate utilization, and changing technology or practice patterns influence demand. These make the accurate projection of demand more difficult.

In the following, *need* will used to refer to the services that ought to be consumed, and *demand* will refer to the services that are or will be consumed. While the need and demand distinction is important, as a practical matter, many methods take into account elements of both. The planner should be aware of this as he both selects and uses any particular method.

CRITERIA FOR EVALUATING METHODS

What factors should be considered in choosing a method for determining the need or demand for health services? Brown *et al.* in their monograph, *Methods for Hospital Services and Bed Need Assessment* suggest four considerations—validity, reliability, accuracy, and complexity.[6]

Validity refers to the ability of a method or technique to measure what it purports to measure. The planner or administrator must ask whether a particular technique incorporates the variables which are considered to influence significantly the quantity of services or beds required. Demographic factors and past and current utilization are obvious examples.

Reliability is the consistency or dependability of the method and is a function of the kinds of data used in the assessment technique. Morbidity data of common contagious diseases, for instance, is a good example of data that are generally considered unreliable. This is due to the fact that many individuals with common ailments do not seek medical care either because they do not consider a particular illness serious or do not translate their felt need into demand. In either case, morbidity data derived from physician reports would not be very reliable.

Accuracy is closely related to validity and reliability and is a measure of the degree to which the output of a method predicts the actual experience the method is designed to measure or predict. The accuracy of a method may be difficult to document because of the effect that supply has on demand. The notion that supply creates its own demand or a "bed built is a bed filled" is now widely accepted in health planning and makes conclusions about accuracy difficult.[7] The better a method is in predicting the future, however, the more valuable it will be.

Finally, *complexity* of a method in and of itself should be considered. The complexity of a method should not necessarily be associated with its ability to assess service requirements. Complexity both increases the difficulty of explaining a method and adds to its cost. On the other hand, a method should not be avoided simply because it is complex. A method should be chosen in light of its costs, required staff capability, and expected results.

It is important also to consider the answers to several questions which address a method's capabilities before selecting it for use.

1. *Does the method provide for the specification of the population whose service requirements are to be determined?* For each service the population dependent upon it may vary. For example, only those under 16 or so are potentially the service population for pediatric care. The size of the population dependent on a given service and their likelihood of requiring it is an important consideration for any method.

2. *Does the method identify, measure, and predict the occurrences in the population that warrant the need for services?* Illness, accidents, and disability produce the need for certain services. In order to measure and predict the extent of need, a method must identify and analyze the occurrence of such circumstances in the population. The extent of such conditions projected into the future and the corresponding set of services that ought to be utilized represent a target for planning and development of resources.

3. *Does the method predict the type and amount of utilization or demand that will occur?* Whatever the extent of need, the planner's first concern is that resources are adequate in order to meet the demand which actually will occur in the future. Some methods focus directly on predicting utilization.

4. *Does the method consider the appropriateness of utilization or demand?* Methods may measure and analyze existing patterns or trends of utilization as a basis for predicting the future, without an attempt to evaluate whether such utilization should be perpetrated. Others may prescribe what utilization ought to be compared to some standard or benchmark. Still others may critically examine actual utilization to determine what utilization ought to occur.

5. *Does the method specify the type and amount of resources required to provide the services that will be utilized?* Some methods will consider the resources, e.g. facilities, beds, manpower, and equipment that are required. In a sense, this is the bottom line since planning and regulatory decisions will focus most on resources requirements.

6. *Does the method consider resource capacity and productivity?* Just as current utilization may or may not be appropriate, a resource's capacity and productivity may be more or less optimal. A method can require consideration or provide judgements about these factors prior to producing estimates of resource requirements.

As several methods are described in the next section, reference will be made to these questions and an attempt made to assess how each method responds to them. Five categories of methods will be discussed and a specific example of a method which represents each category will be described.

There is no concensus of the typology which is most useful for organizing methods. The one chosen here uses the general statistical technique employed in the method as the basis for classification. The categories of methods which will be discussed include the formula approach, the regression approach, the stochastic approach, simulation, and the ratio approach.

METHOD A: THE FORMULA APPROACH

Description

Because of its simplicity and its past use by the Hill-Burton agencies as a basis for determining how to allocate health facility construction funds, the formula is perhaps the most widely used method for determining bed requirements. The basic formula projects future utilization by multiplying the current use rate by projected population. It is ordinarily given as a segmented set of formulas:

$$\frac{\text{current patient-days}}{\text{current population}} = \text{use rate}$$

$$\frac{(\text{use rate}) \ (\text{projected population})}{365} = \text{average daily census}$$

$$\frac{\text{average daily census}}{\text{desired occupancy rate}} = \text{projected beds required}$$

If the current population of an area were 1,000,000 and total patient-days were 800,000, then the use rate would be:

$$\frac{800,000 \text{ patient-days}}{1,000,000 \text{ people}} = .8$$

If the projected population for 1980 were 1.2 million, then future utilization would be estimated as:

$$(.8) \times (1,200,000) = 960,000 \text{ patient-days}$$

Average daily census is determined by dividing this by the number of days in a year:

$$\frac{960,000}{365} = 2,630$$

This figure is then divided by a desired occupancy rate, for example, 85 percent:

$$\frac{2630}{.85} = 3094 \text{ projected beds required}$$

This is an estimate of the total beds required to serve the projected 1980 population.

This formula approach thus sets up a relationship between beds required and population; as population changes, so do bed requirements. Much criticism has been made of this simple approach. Some of the deficiencies can be overcome by making adjustments to the formula as described below.

Utilization Adjustment

One simple adjustment in the above can be made that will allow for a change in the use rate in addition to a change in population. By analyzing past utilization, a trend of past use can be determined. If, for example, the use rate is declining at a rate of one percent per year, then the projection for five years would include an adjustment as follows.

$$\text{Future use rate} = \text{current use rate} \times \left(1 \text{ minus } [(\text{rate of change}) \times (\text{number of years in the projection})]\right)$$

$$= .8 \times \left(1 - [(.01) \times (5 \text{ years})]\right)$$

$$= .8 \times (1 - .05)$$

$$= .8 \times .95 = .76$$

$$\text{Future utilization} = 1,200,000 \times .76$$
$$= 912,000 \text{ patient-days}$$

$$\text{ADC} = \frac{912,000}{365} = 2499$$

$$\text{Beds required} = \frac{2499}{.85} = 2939$$

One hundred and fifty-five less beds are required as a result of this expected decrease in utilization.

Service Type Adjustment

Another type of adjustment that can be made recognizes the specific types of hospital bed units. Separate utilization rates may be determined for each type of service (medical, surgical, obstetric, pediatric), and projections may be made accordingly. In addition to identifying separate use rates, the adjustment recognizes that occupancy levels may vary for each separate service. Higher occupancy levels are more commonly achieved for medical/surgical services than for obstetric or pediatric services.

Patient Origin Adjustment

A third adjustment to the formula can be made so that persons outside the area may be explicitly included. To accomplish this, patient origin data must be collected to separate the utilization of services by people outside the area. Different use rates can then be assigned to this population if it is warranted. The formula recognizing utilization of an area's services by persons living within and outside of the area is:

$U = (a \times b) + (c \times d \times e)$, where:

U = utilization expressed as total patient-days per year for some future year.

a = population of the area from which that utilization originated for the same future year.

b = adjusted use rate (patient-days per thousand) for the HSA population only as projected for the future year.

c = measured admissions of persons living outside the area.

d = average length of stay.

e = expected change in utilization by those from outside the area.

Age/Sex Adjustment

Utilization rates can be measured and predicted on an age/sex cohort basis. Since only children use pediatric beds, the utilization rate should be measured as pediatric patient-days divided by the pediatric population. Future utilization should then be predicted on the basis of the future population changes within this age group. Obstetric utilization, for example, can be estimated by determining the number of women of the child-bearing age and the fertility rate. If the annual fertility rate is anticipated to be 75 per 1,000 for 1980, for example, this figure may be a basis for predicting obstetric utilization by applying that rate to the 1980 population of women from ages 15 to 44. Some further adjustment would be needed to account for obstetric utilization other than delivery. Accuracy can, thus, be further improved by dividing the population into cohorts and measuring and projecting utilization for each age/sex group.

Appropriateness Adjustment

Some analysis of the nature of the utilization currently experienced can be undertaken. If inpatient utilization is very high, then future utilization review designed to decrease inappropriate utilization or the development of alternatives to hospitalization such as long term and ambulatory care may result in significant reduction in the utilization of hospital care. If such a reduction can and will be achieved, future hospital development should be geared to these projected utilization levels. Alternatively, utilization may be low, and there may be evidence that there are significant financial or other barriers to care (e.g. a low percentage of the population has insurance coverage). In this case, the probability of this situation's changing (e.g. increase in insurance coverage) should be considered and its effect on utilization predicted.

A detailed methodology for assessing the appropriateness of utilization has been developed and carried out in Rochester, New York by the Genesee Regional Health Planning Council.[8] While this is described as a way to adjust the formula, its usefulness extends beyond this for planning purposes, and it can be used as input to adjust other methods described as well.

The objective of this method is to estimate the population's need for various levels of care. Since that population should be composed of persons in facilities and persons judged to require acute care services, defining the inpatient population is a long, concentrated effort, involving numerous information sources. In Rochester, visiting nurses from the local health department and the voluntary visiting nurse agency identified persons requiring such institutional care. A mail survey, endorsed by the local medical society, was used to ask physicians to identify anyone they thought should be receiving institutional care. Local social service agencies, church groups, letter carriers, and others assisted in identifying persons suspected of needing inpatient care. Television and radio were also used to generate more information on patient information. The result of all this data gathering was a master list of names with duplicate entries eliminated.[9]

Physician-nurse teams surveyed both the institutionalized and the noninstitutionalized persons identified. Judgements were recorded as to what services were needed by each person and what level of care could best provide those services. This method results in an overall estimate of need as opposed to demand for services. The most appropriate levels of care for all persons surveyed were identified, and an estimate of inappropriate utilization was developed.

Desired Occupancy Adjustment

Finally, occupancy levels related to hospital size can be used to translate expected utilization into bed requirements. Isolating utilization by service with different occupancy standards for each as suggested above is a start, but the actual variation in utilization would be a better guide than an arbitrary standard for determining beds required. In the case where there is a large number of existing beds with fairly stable utilization levels, 90 percent occupancy or greater can probably be achieved. In cases where the number of beds is small and there is great variation in utilization, 50 or 60 percent occupancy may be viewed as satisfactory. A method for determining desired occupancy under different risk conditions is presented under Method C, the Stochastic Approach.

Discussion

The basic bed-need formula, excluding the adjustments which have been discussed, has a number of major limitations. The formula focuses solely on demand, and the major variable affecting it is its population. It assumes that the future patient population will utilize the facility in the same manner as the current population. As such, the validity of the formula will depend on the nature of the region to which it is applied. It will be more valid, and in turn more accurate, in areas that remain demographically stable, such as rural areas, and is best used for short term projections of service and facility requirements. Its major advantage is that it is not complex and the data it requires is readily available.

Only three of the questions discussed earlier can be answered positively when looking at the basic formula. The formula approach is based on a specific population, projects future demand based on changes in that population, and specifies the number of beds required. If the adjustments described are made, then other of the questions raised can be answered positively or more completely.

The age/sex and patient-origin adjustments can be used to better define the population for which planning is to be undertaken. This should lead to better judgements about required services and resources because the demographic factors which cause differences in utilization are recognized.

The appropriateness adjustment provides for an estimate of the services needed. Without it, no attention is paid to the possibility that there may be persons in the population who should be, but are not, using services and there is no questioning of the appropriateness of current utilization. If current utilization levels include significant amounts of improper utilization, the situation will tend to be perpetuated by the basic formula. It is important to point out that the appropriateness adjustment as described is based on a one-time or cross-sectional sample and that some estimate of its reliability is needed as a basis for generalizing about appropriateness over a period of time.

Accuracy in projecting utilization can be improved with the utilization adjustment, which recognizes and accounts for changes in the use rate. Without it, the formula assumes that future utilization rates will be identical to those of the past. Thus, the formula can be improved by making adjustments to it. While some of the adjustments cancel out one of the method's primary advantages—its simplicity—the adjustments can serve to improve estimates of future bed requirements.

METHOD B— THE REGRESSION APPROACH

Description

Regression is a technique in which independent variables are incorporated into an equation to extrapolate a value for a dependent variable such as patient-days, admissions, visits, etc.[10] This is stated in the general case as $Y = a + bx$ where x is the independent variable and Y is the dependent variable. Such an equation can use one or more independent variables to predict the dependent variable.

Two forms of regression are most likely to be used for analysis:

1. $Y = a + b_1 x_1 + b_2 x_2 + \ldots b_n x_n$

OR

2. $Y = ax_1^{b_1} x_2^{b_2} \ldots x_n^{b_n}$

The first form is the standard multiple linear regression form where Y (visits or admissions) is predicted on a basis of a constant (a) plus the effects of each variable (x) weighted by coefficient (b). The second form is an exponential rather than linear approach where Y is the product of a constant (a) times each of the variables (x) weighted by an exponent (b).

In determining appropriate values for the constants, coefficients, or exponents, past utilization is analyzed in terms of the collected values for each of the input variables. Since this is a complex process, it may be necessary to rely on both personnel experienced with regression analysis and a computer. A stepwise approach (adding each variable one at a time) will identify the variables most highly correlated with differences in utilization. Variables with little or no predictive ability may be deleted from the analysis.

The regression approach can be used to predict the utilization for any type of health services provided adequate historical data on the independent and dependent variables are available. To emphasize this, an outpatient rather than an inpatient example is described below. This specific method was developed to predict the expected utilization of outpatient services (expressed in patient visits) for a rural population in a given future year.[11] This model has been applied in Georgia and assumes that demand for service arises from two basic processes. First, the incidence of dysfunction generates a need, and second, this need is translated into demand. There are three general aspects of the need to demand translation. First, the knowledge, attitude, and expectation of the individual (and possibly of the immediate family) determines whether the dysfunction is considered worthy and amenable to treatment. Second, the availability of health care and its costs are considered. Finally, the financial resources available to the individual must be compared to the expected costs of the services.[12] Based on this, four types of factors were identified to predict ambulatory care visits: demographic, sociological, economic, and health supply variables (see Table 5-1).

In order to use the method, past experience of ambulatory care resources was obtained. Characteristics of the service population and attributes of the health system serving that population were determined. The information concerning the four factors was then analyzed as independent variables in the regression analysis. The analysis resulted in the identification of variables which best explained the variation in utilization and the assignment of weights or coefficients to each. The resulting equation might then read:

annual per capita rate of outpatient visits = .325 + .0003 (per capital income) + .0002 (average cost of a hospital day) − .154 (cumulative fertility rate) + 3.95 (ratio of individual age less than 15 to total population). . . .

Discussion

It is difficult to discuss the characteristics of the regression method without talking about a specific application, as in the example. One caveat is important. There is often a tendency to infer a causal relationship between variables included in the regression equation and the dependent variable—demand for visits or hospital admissions. The regression equation, however, does not necessarily suggest cause and effect between demand and the factors influencing demand.[13] The independent variables were included in the equation because they were highly correlated with a historical pattern of demand, not because they caused it.

The regression approach should be fairly valid since many variables can be included. However, some studies utilizing a regression model have found that its forecasting power is no better than a relatively straightforward formula technique.[14] Regression tends to be less effective under rapidly changing conditions. The longer the time frame to be forecast, the less accurate the result is likely to be. It is also important that the population being planned for be accurately identified initially, or the variables included in the regression equation will misrepresent the actual population and result in an inaccurate prediction of demand. This approach is relatively complex as it requires a computer and someone knowledgeable about the use of regressional analysis. To develop an adequate equation, a large number of variables may need to be examined. This will affect the amount of data required and the time and cost of the analysis.

TABLE 5-1
EXAMPLE INDEPENDENT VARIABLES FOR REGRESSION EQUATION

1. Population characteristics:
   — Ratio of four age categories to total population (less than 15, 15 to 44, 45 to 64, 65 and over)
   — Ratio of white population to total population
   — Cumulative fertility rate for women 35 to 44

2. Sociological variables
   — Percent of families with children under 6
   — Median school years completed—persons 25 and over
   — Percent migrants

3. Economic variables
   — Average cost of a visit to an outpatient clinic
   — Percent unemployed
   — Per capita income

4. Health supply variables
   — Ratio of general beds to total population
   — Ratio of general practice physicians to total population
   — Rate of admissions to general hospital

Source: Frederic D. Kennedy, "Macro Econometric Model of the Demand for Ambulatory Health Services." Paper presented at the Symposium on Methods for Determining and Projecting Need and Demand for Ambulatory Services, sponsored by BHRD, HEW, May 19-21, 1975, p.3.

Turning to the specific example, it describes a certain service population but does not specifically address the circumstances under which ambulatory services will be utilized. Morbidity, trauma, or disease levels of the population are not determined, although demographic factors that might affect these levels are included. Since utilization experience is used to develop the regression, that experience is accepted uncritically and its appropriateness is not assessed, although adjustments could be made for this. While the method does predict utilization or demand, it does not provide for its conversion to resource requirements.

The relative advantages and disadvantages of this method hinge on whether a reliable regression equation can be developed and whether accurate projections can be made of future variables that go into it. This method is certainly more costly (ten times or more) and requires greater specialized expertise than the bed need formula.

One of the greatest potential uses of this method may lie in its usefulness as a simulator rather than a predictor. If variables are chosen for the equation that can be altered deliberately in the future, the regression may be used to identify changes necessary to achieve a desired future rather than merely to predict a likely one. If a target utilization level could be identified (by using another method), the regression method might identify how that utilization target might be achieved. Thus, the level of demand that would best serve a specified population's needs and insure efficient use of resources might be identified and possibly achieved.

METHOD C: THE STOCHASTIC APPROACH

Description

A number of methods that are used to determine bed need are based on probability theory. These techniques are based on assumptions about the arrival and discharge process of the hospital or outpatient facility and, in essence, attempt to match that specific process with a special statistical technique. For example, the Poisson distribution assumes that arrivals to a hospital are random but occur at a certain average rate. Queueing theory can then be applied as a representation of how patients will arrive and wait for admission.[15] The application of such stochastic methods has primarily taken place at the institutional level, which differentiates them from many of the other approaches discussed.

The method chosen as an example of this approach addresses the problem of translating expected utilization into bed requirements.[16] It offers a statistical basis for such a translation that is different than applying average occupancy rates to calculate bed requirements as is characteristic of the formula approach. Instead of using averages, this method examines patterns of fluctuation in hospital census and prescribes bed requirements based on predictions of the probability that census will reach or exceed a given level. Thus, its objective is to determine the minimum number of beds needed by services at a hospital to alleviate high occupancy rates and excessive waiting time without creating future excess bed capacity. The information required for this method includes expected utilization of hospital beds by service (pediatric,

FIGURE 5-1
DISTRIBUTION OF DAILY CENSUS PEDIATRICS

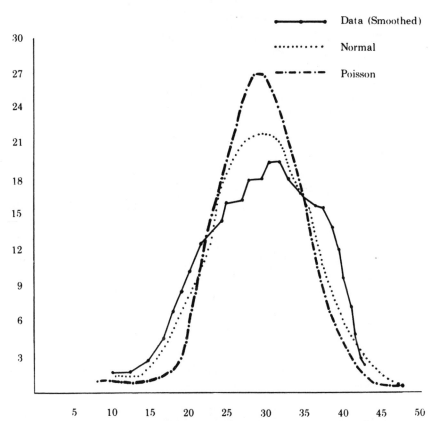

Source: Richard DuFour, "Planning for Acute Inpatient Services—A Probabilistic Model for Relating the Determination of Bed Requirements to the Level of Services to be Provided." Paper presented at Symposium on Methods for Determining and Projecting Need and Demand for Inpatient Services sponsored by BHPRD, HEW, February 3-5, 1975, p. 7.

obstetric, medical/surgical) and data concerning the fluctuations in demand for each type of care. Deliberate choices can be made as to the risk one is willing to take that on a given day there may be a greater demand than the number of beds available.

In applying this method, the actual census level of an institution is first examined. A frequency distribution is then prepared indicating the number of times each year a census level is reached. The pattern is likely to be that of the bell-shaped curve. This is compared with that which would have been predicted by Poisson and normal distribution. Figure 5-1 indicates a fairly close fit between actual data and what would have been predicted by the Poisson and normal distribution, with the normal distribution a slightly better fit. This finding is important because of the predictability of occurrences of the normal distribution. Once the standard deviation of the average census has been determined, one can predict variation from the average data census (ADC) with a high degree of certainty. For example, only two and a half percent of the time will the census be higher than two standard deviations above the ADC. If one is willing to accept that nine days a year (two and a half percent) the demand for beds may exceed capacity, then the beds required may be set at expected ADC plus 1.96 times its standard deviation.

If, for example, ADC is 100 and the standard deviation is determined to be 10 (standard deviation under the Poisson/normal distribution is equal to the square root of the mean), bed requirements can be calculated. To meet expected demands on all but nine days a year, 120 beds would be required—that is, ADC and $1.96\sqrt{ADC}$ or $100 + 1.96 (10)$. To be sure of having enough beds 99 percent of the time, or all but approximately four days a year, 123 beds would be required. Thus, the result of using this method will be an estimate of the number of beds needed to accommodate demand under whatever risk of shortage is chosen. Such a shortage in those few cases, when it occurs, might be handled by referring or transferring patients to other institutions or by going above 100 percent occupancy by using space not normally used for beds.

Discussion

This method addresses only a part of the need or demand determination process, that of translating some expected level of utilization into bed requirements. It does not help in predicting future utilization, and, as such, it must be used in conjunction with another method. Compared to the bed need formula, this method will call for fewer total beds whenever the expected daily census is a reasonably large number. It also allows for explicit consideration of the risk of shortage. At an expected census of 400, for example, this method using a 97.5 percent risk level would result in a requirement for 439 beds (400 + 1.96 × 20). This would yield an occupancy rate of 91 percent, one significantly higher than that used as the usual formula standard (85 percent). An 81-bed hospital using the same risk factor would yield an 82 percent occupancy. Thus, as the number of beds decreases, so will the target occupancy using this approach.

A major problem with this method is that of validity. Unless the average census is normally distributed and expected to remain so, this method has questionable validity. While samples of observations have shown that the normal distribution describes the ADC as in the example used, there is not a solid theoretical basis for stating that this relationship will hold in all situations.[17] One of the other weaknesses of the stochastic approaches, given the regional nature of many planning problems, is that they are most applicable at the institutional level. If one could assume that there is a common queue for all of the institutions in a community—that is, there are no preferences for individual institutions and physicians had admitting privileges to all institutions—then the method could be applied to a group of hospitals. This could result in achieving high occupancy since a large number of beds would be involved. However, in very few communities could one accept the underlying assumptions.

METHOD D — SIMULATION

Description

Simulation involves the development of a model that describes the behavior of a system. It is a representation of a system and how it operates. It is usually composed of a series of measurable events which can be allowed to interact under different conditions to generate different results.[18] One such model has been developed by the Texas Hospital Association.[19] The model quantitatively portrays the health care delivery system as it exists and is specifically designed to permit changes in the system. Its objective is to predict the demand for care in terms of ambulatory care visits, inpatient admissions, and patient-days for specific geographic areas. These predictions can then be converted into the number of beds required to supply the predicted demand.

This simulation requires two major types of information: data on the service population in terms of factors affecting utilization and data on health system factors. As the model was originally applied, it included the following:

1. Total population
2. Population divided into eleven age cohorts

3. Per capita income
4. Average household income
5. Percentage of households with income over $10,000
6. Number of physicians
7. Average hospital size
8. Total number of hospital beds
9. Average nursing home size
10. Percent of population under 65 with health insurance
11. Public expenditures for health care[20]

Data on these variables were collected for a twelve-year period (1960-1972) for the nine census divisions in the United States. In addition, actual utilization data of hospital and outpatient care was acquired.

The simulation attempts to describe the interactions between the population served and its health system. Prediction equations were developed using multiple regression analysis. Actual utilization data from the past was used as the dependent variable while the population and health system characteristics were used as independent variables. Because of the complexity of the simulation and the large amount of data required, a computer is necessary.

The output of the simulation is an estimate of future utilization of acute inpatient care under certain conditions. By including predicted change in population and other demographic variables, the simulation will predict what future system utilization is likely to be. By making changes in the health system characteristics, for example, the number may be evaluated and a deliberate course of action may be developed to achieve rather than merely predict a future level of utilization. Similarly, given a desired utilization level, the output could be the set of health system changes that would achieve it.

To implement the model in a given geographic area, several validation steps are required to insure close agreement between the model's outputs and historical observations. The model can then be refined to reflect more closely that observation and improve its accuracy.

Discussion

One of the major advantages of the simulation model is its ability to be used to study or evaluate different strategies and courses of action without disrupting the system. This becomes important in evaluating different courses of action. As such, the simulation, which makes use of the other models discussed, such as regression, is more flexible than most other methods. This model, however, is much more complex and expensive and requires specialized expertise to use. For this reason, the simulation is perhaps more helpful in looking at the effects of major and complex projected changes in the system, such as the passage of national health insurance, than in making the more routine projections of need or demand for services.

The specific example described may be applied to almost any identified service population. It focuses on demand and does not address appropriate utilization of services or need for services. Similarly, it does not directly specify the number or types of resources required. However, since the number of available beds is one of the input factors in the simulation itself, the effect of different numbers of beds on utilization could be determined.

Although assumptions are made in a simulation model, the design of the model probably requires greater explicitness about those assumptions than other methods. Care must be taken to examine these assumptions to assure they correspond to the reality of the situation to which they are about to be applied. This may require considerable study of that situation. Because of its cost and complexity, simulation models, as they have been developed to date, will probably not be practical for use in most planning settings.

METHOD E — THE RATIO APPROACH

Description

Ratio methods establish simple quantitative relationships between two variables. While not as widely used in facility planning, the ratio method is the traditional and most widely used method for estimating health manpower requirements. Planners use this method to characterize the current manpower situation, to assess the adequacy of the present health manpower supply, and to determine the number of personnel that will be required to provide the community with health services in the future that are equivalent to a national, regional, minimal, or optimal level.[21] The assumption underlying the manpower/population ratio is that population is the major determinant of manpower requirements.

This method is much less useful in facility planning because of the difficulty in establishing a meaningful ratio. In addition to the relationships between beds and population, another important influence on bed requirements is hospital size, as has been indicated. The larger the hospital, the lower its bed to population ratio is likely to be. This has led to a wide variation in current bed to population ratios. For example, the average ratio of beds per 1,000 persons ranges from 6.9 in North Dakota to 3.0 in Maryland.[22] For these reasons, the bed to population ratio is not likely to be useful for planning and regulatory decisions.

A more complex method building on the ratio approach, however, is worth describing. This method sets up relationships between age/sex cohorts and mortality estimates, and then relationships between morbidity and service requirements. It has been applied specifically to the state of California and employs a broad conceptual model of the health system to determine health needs of a given population.[23] The information used in carrying out this method includes the demographic characteristics of a specific population. Estimates of morbidity levels in that population must then be made to be identified by the International Standard Classification of Diseases. Based on these estimates, determinations are made of the type and amount of services required. Each service is characterized by the type of provider who renders it. By totalling all the service requirements for the entire population, total service requirements can be determined.

There are a number of different approaches which can be used for translating estimated morbidity into service needs. Individual panels of experts with consumer input might determine services needed for each average case of each diagnosis included in the morbidity estimates. An alternative to this approach would be to study a known population believed to receive high quality medical care and determine the average services per diagnosis actually received. The method as applied originally, employed the latter approach. The population chosen as a basis for planning was the entire population of the state of California. Estimates of morbidity expected in this population were derived from a study of insurance claims by Group Health Insurance, Inc. of New York, covering its 1964 experience. The reported morbidity among the populations served by GHI was isolated by age/sex categories, and morbidity rates were separated by diagnosis. These rates were applied to the 1970 California population to estimate its morbidity. The actual experience of GHI subscribers in 1964 was then used to convert morbidity into service requirements. For example, a review of the data shows that the rates of diagnosis for infective and parasitic diseases per 1,000 population was 184.4 cases per 1,000 for males under five years of age. By applying this and other expected morbidity rates to the appropriate age/sex cohort, the total number of cases of this diagnosis can be computed. Then, this figure is multiplied by a service ratio to get the expected number of hospital admissions office visits, laboratory tests, etc. The output of this method is the total hospital admissions (or other service requirement) one could expect to occur based on morbidity and service ratios used as standards.

This can be converted into resource requirements using other methods which have been described, e.g., the "bed need' formula.

Discussion

The simplicity of the general ratio method is its greatest advantage. Relative to other methods, the physician or bed-to-population ratio requires minimal data, can be quickly calculated at low cost, and requires modest staff expertise. It is useful as a descriptive device, as input to more sophisticated methods, and as validation of estimates derived by other means.[24]

The weaknesses of the method are, however, great. Changes in the future involving socioeconomic conditions, technological advance, and alteration of practice patterns or the delivery system are ignored, although they will affect demand. The general ratio method for facility planning has the added weakness of not considering fluctuations in demand and hospital size as a determinant of bed requirements. The specific example discussed is far more useful than the general ratio. It identifies a specific population for which planning is to be undertaken. More important, it specifically examines the conditions under which hospital inpatient care is likely to be required. As such, it comes closer than the other methods discussed in measuring need.

Objections may be raised to the example cited because it used Group Health Insurance, Inc. (GHI) data. Being old, the data may not be representative of the situation some ten years later. Since the data are specific to a population in New York who are covered by GHI, they may not be typical of other populations. The data represent only cases diagnosed and treated by GHI physicians and do not account for members' use of non-GHI physicians.

The method also converts morbidity into expected health service utilization and isolates hospital utilization by major services. But, since in the example service utilization is also based on 1964 GHI data, additional problems arise. For example, service utilization is initially based on the extent of GHI members' awareness of a health problem. Such awareness may not be typical of other populations. Subsequent service utilization is a physician's determination, and GHI physicians may not be typical of other physicians. Finally, the data were collected prior to the Medicare and Medicaid legislation and subsequent changes in utilization among the aged and poor populations.

If actual morbidity levels for a population and better estimates of service requirements could be developed from local experience, the objections above would not apply. In this case, however, the rates or standards for converting morbidity into service requirements may not yield valid predictions since it does not necessarily represent the utilization that will occur. It may well be that the expected morbidity will occur, but that not all people suffering from a specific condition will behave according to the standard.

Although this method does not propose a conversion formula for translating expected utilization into bed requirements, it provides a basis—hospital admissions—for doing so. Since utilization is isolated by services, the data are more useful than if only total utilization were addressed. However, before developing hospital construction plans based on this method, the planner will want to assure himself that the projected utilization levels will occur or can be made to occur.

SUMMARY COMPARISON OF METHODS

To compare the various capabilities and weaknesses of the example methods described, Table 5-2 has been developed. It summarizes points in the discussion by answering the questions that were presented earlier. It should be pointed out that the five-part typology used to describe the methods for determining need is far from exact. In essence, the major factor used to distinguish the different groups is the statistical method or approach used. Since some of the examples used more than one statistical method, their placement in a group may be somewhat arbitrary.

From the descriptions of the methods presented, it should be readily apparent that there is no "best method." Depending on the population for which planning is undertaken and its characteristics, the characteristics of the health system, and the resources and capabilities of those responsible for planning, one or another of the methods will be evaluated as most appropriate. To answer satisfactorily all of the questions raised as criteria for evaluating methods, some combination of methods will, in most cases, be needed.

THE PLANNING PROCESS

It is important that any method for determining need be used as part of an overall planning process. It is not the purpose here to detail a process since they are very well described in many other places. The American Hospital Association, for example, suggests a nine-step process:

1. Define the area of need/issue
2. Analyze the area of need/issue
3. Define general goals related to need/issue

4. Set specific objectives
5. Identify alternative courses of action
6. Select desired alternative courses of action
7. Develop a specific course of action
8. Implement course of action
9. Evaluate[25]

The methods which have been discussed relate most to steps 1 and 2.

While it is important that each hospital engage in planning on an institutional basis, it is equally important that institutions participate and support the community and area-wide planning processes established by PL 93-641. From that involvement can come an understanding of community characteristics and health problems, a knowledge of the health planning efforts of others, and a better appreciation of the resources, e.g., population data and staff expertise, which the HSA may be able to make available to facilitate institutional planning.

At either the HSA or institutional level, need determination and the other steps of the planning process must be carried out with careful attention to what are politically acceptable solutions. Planning implies change, and plans must be designed in such a way as to create actions which are implementable. Similarly, any plan developed reflects the values of those who have prepared it. Such values may or may not be explicit but will certainly influence the planning process from the choice of methods to the design of specific actions for resolving problems. A situation may develop where a solution may not be acceptable to all participants in a planning process because values are not clear. If participants' values and orientation can be made explicit, some agreement on the planning process and its outcome is more likely.

Understanding the environment and the trends affecting health care is an important part of this process. A growing and future dominant trend is the concern over rapidly rising health care costs and the growing percentage of resources which the United States is allocating for health care. Such will surely have implications for the planning process and perhaps influence the choice of planning methods. An example of this trend as related to need determination methods is contained in the following response by Dr. Paul Elwood to a recent review of such methods, which for the most part have focused on the demand for hospital beds.

The majority of bed need criteria that planning agencies intend to use simply keep one step ahead of the demand created by a growing health care market fueled by the inflationary pull of advances in technology and the push of expanding third-party

Table 5-2
COMPARISON OF METHODS USED IN DETERMINING NEED

Criteria Questions	A Formula Method	B Regression Method	C Stochastic Method	D Simulation	E Ratio Method
1. Does the method provide for the specification of the population whose service requirements are to be determined?	Based on population of political jurisdictions; patient origin adjustment can help refine	Based on the Number of persons who have been using hospital beds in an area in the past	No	Can be used for any population; accepts factors for adjusting the population	Can be used for any area or population characteristics provided the data is available
2. Does the method identify, measure, and predict the occurrence in the population that warrants the *need* for services?	No, addresses only demand or utilization; appropriateness adjustment brings estimate closer to need	No, addresses only demand or utilization, not those who need but don't receive care	No	No, past utilization used to determine future demand	Yes, specifically addresses by estimating population mobility
3. Does the method predict the type and amount of utilization or *demand* that will occur?	Yes, straight line projection of past utilization	Yes	No	Yes, addresses expected utilization under different circumstances	Yes, predicts utilization by major service although there is less certainty that utilization will occur

4. Does the method consider the appropriateness of utilization or demand?	The basic method does not address; the appropriateness adjustment does	Accepts past utilization	No	Accepts current utilization	No, does not consider except in the standard that might be set to translate morbidity to service requirements
5. Does the method specify the type and amount of resources required to provide the service that will be utilized?	Uses target occupancy to translate utilization to bed requirements	Service levels predicted, but does not produce resource requirements	Translate expected utilization into bed requirements by type of service	Resource requirements not specifically addressed	Service levels established, but does not produce resource requirements
6. Does the method consider resource capacity or productivity?	Uses occupancy standard, e.g. 85%	No	Specifically addresses by considering risk of all beds being full	Does not consider, but the simulation can be used to test the effects of different capacities	No

coverage. Criteria of this type may protect the planning agency from legal attacks and most certainly will give the planning process an aura of quantitative objectivity. But, for what limited objective? Preventing duplication of facilities, or perhaps making it easier to decide who will get new facilities, but at the risk of rationalizing continuing medical inflation by giving community pseudoscientific sanction to health facilities that sustain demand at already higher than necessary levels.

Roemer's observation that extra beds stimulate extra hospitalization has been used as an important rationale for publicly controlling the supply of hospital beds. How can we conceivably use bed supply to control use if the demand for beds is used as the criteria for establishing the optimal supply of beds? [26]

He goes on to say that planning should be aimed at reducing the supply of beds and suggests that the reduction takes place to such an extent that the bed supply should play a rationalizing role.

In support of this line of thinking are recent studies that document wide variation in age-adjusted incidence of surgery. A study of service areas in Maine, for example, showed a nearly three-fold difference in surgery rates for nine common surgical procedures.[27] The conclusion of this study suggests that this difference occurs because of differences in opinion among physicians concerning the effectiveness of specific treatments or differences in the way physicians define health care needs.[28] The planner is beginning to have to ask "should planning project such differences in utilization into the future and encourage the building of additional facilities to handle them?" Each institution and, in turn, each community planning process must answer this question and consider the response in light of other important issues and trends. These might include the desire to increase accessibility to care, continuity and acceptability concerns, and efforts to maintain or increase quality of care. The methods for determining service and facility requirements described are thus only partially helpful in arriving at planning solutions.

CRITERIA AND STANDARDS FOR REVIEW

In addition to the output of a planning process and the resultant Health Systems Plan and Annual Implementation plan, the Health Systems Agency and the State Health Planning and Development Agency will develop and adopt standards and criteria which will probably broaden the factors used in reviewing requests under CON and 1122 review processes. PL 93-641, Section 1532(c) requires the consideration of at least the following criteria:

1. The relationship of the health services being reviewed to the applicable HSP and AIP

2. The relationship of services reviewed to the long-range development plan (if any) of the persons providing or proposing such services

3. The need that the population served or to be served by such services has for such services

4. The availability of alternative, less costly, or more effective methods of providing such services

5. The relationship of services reviewed to the existing health care system of the area in which such services are provided or proposed to be provided

6. In the case of health services proposed to be provided, the availability of resources (including health manpower, management personnel, and funds for capital and operating needs) for the provision of such services and the availability of alternative uses of such resources for the provision of other health services

7. The special needs and circumstances of those entitites which provide a substantial portion of their services or resources, or both, to individuals not residing in the health service areas in which the entities are located or in adjacent health service areas (such entities may include medical and other professional schools, multidisciplinary clinics, specialty centers, and other entities as the secretary may by regulation prescribe)

8. The special needs and circumstances of HMOs for which assistance may be provided under Title XIII

9. In the case of a constructive project—
    a. the costs and methods of the proposed construction, and
    b. the probable impact of the construction project reviewed on the costs of providing health services by the person proposing such construction projects

Health providers will have to take these and other criteria adopted by the HSA governing body into account when they seek approval for proposals requiring reviews under CON or 1122. Institutional providers must pay especially close attention to criterion 1 (its proposal's relationship to the HSP/AIP), 2 (its proposal's relationship to its own institution's long range plan), 3 (the population's need for the proposal's services), and 4 (how the proposal's services fit into and are coordinated with existing medical services). Although the methods for determining a population's need or demand for services are mainly geared to the planning of a HSA, the data developed, the criterion and standards used and the plan created by the HSA using these methods should be helpful to and serve as the basis for the institutional provider's development of its own plan, and the medical care proposals related to it. In this way, the institutional provider can develop its own proposals in the most expeditious and least costly manner and at the same time provide the HSA and SA review bodies with a basis for fairly evaluating the proposal against the region's and state's plans.

SUMMARY AND CONCLUSIONS

Planning requires that some description of the future be developed both as it is likely to be, given no specific intervention, and as it might be if specific actions are initiated. Such forecasts require the analysis of past and current trends and the use of judgement about how such trends are likely to change or can be influenced. The mechanical use of any of the methods described will lead to unsatisfactory results. Judgement also has to be used in considering and selecting a method for determining service and facility requirements building in consideration of available resources for planning, levels of sophistication required, population characteristics, the current status of the health care delivery system, and the political environment and trends affecting it.

Of the five examples provided representing methods that are currently in use, no conclusions can be reached concerning which is best for all situations. Each has certain strengths and weaknesses. None deals explicitly with value questions. Similarly, none clearly considers the impact of changes in technology or weighs issues of cost, acceptability, quality, accessibility, or continuity. Some combination or modification of these or other methods will most likely serve best to meet a particular user's needs. Whatever method is used, it should be used as part of a planning process considering other issues. Much future work is needed to evaluate more critically both the process and outcome of using different methods. In addition, other methods will need to be developed in order to make the increasingly more difficult resource allocation decisions. Planning techniques from other fields need to be studied and their usefulness for health planning evaluated.

Part of the structure for making decisions concerning the services and facilities required by a population is the CON and 1122 processes. Planning, both at the institutional and area-wide levels, provides the basis for the intelligent use of these regulatory mechanisms. The use of appropriate methods for determining health service and facility requirements as part of a planning process will add to the rationality of both planning and regulatory efforts.

Notes

1. Much of the input to this chapter comes from reports prepared for the Bureau of Health Planning and Resources Development, Health Resources Administration, Public Health Service, DHEW. They were based on a series of symposia on methods for determining and projecting needs and demands for health services, which were held early in 1975. The reports were prepared by Arthur Young and Co. under contract HRA 106-74-36. Thomas F. Lantry and Michael B. Harrington, Ph.D. of Arthur Young and Robin E. Mac Stravic, Ph.D. of the Medical College of Virginia played major roles in the preparation of these reports. The author was responsible for the direction of this project.

2. Gordon D. Brown et al., *Methods for Hospital Services and Bed Need Assessment:* A Report to Health Planners and Administrators (University Park, Pa.: Pennsylvania State University, 1975), p. 4.

3. Ibid., p. 6.

4. Sylvester E. Berki, *Hospital Economics* (Lexington: D.C. Heath and Co., 1972), p. 36.

5. Robert M. Crane et al., "The Marketing of Medical Care Services" in *Marketing in the Service Sector,* John M. Rathmell, ed. (Cambridge: Winthrop Publishers, 1974), p. 133.

6. Brown, op. cit., pp. 25-27.

7. M. I. Roemer, "Bed Supply and Hospital Utilization: A National Experiment," *Hospitals* 35 (1961): 36-42.

8. Gloria Haynie and John Hill, "The Method of Estimating Inpatient Bed Needs in the Genesee Region" (Paper presented at the Symposium on Methods for Determining and Projecting Need and Demand for Long Term Care Services, sponsored by the Bureau of health Planning and Resources Development, U.S. Department of Health, Education, and Welfare, November 10-12, 1974), p. 1.

9. Genesee Regional Health Planning Council, *Survey of Need for Inpatient Beds and Related Home Health Services* (Rochester, N.Y.: Genesee Regional Health Planning Council, 1970), p. 1.

10. Brown, op cit., p. 27.

11. Frederick D. Kennedy, "Macro Econometric Model of the Demand for Ambulatory Health Services" (Paper presented at the Symposium on Methods for Determining and Projecting Need and Demand for Ambulatory Services, sponsored by the Bureau of Health Planning and Resources Development, U.S. Department of Health, Education, and Welfare, May 19-21, 1975), p. 1.

12. Ibid., p. 2.

13. Brown, op. cit., p. 28.

14. Carl Hopkins, et al., *Methods of Estimating Hospital Bed Needs* (Los Angeles: University of California Press, 1967), pp. 11-17.

15. Brown, op. cit., p. 34.

16. Richard DuFour, "Planning for Acute Inpatient Services—A Probilistic Model for Relating the Determination of Bed Requirements to the Level of Services to be Provided" (Paper presented at the Symposium on Methods for Determining and Project-

ing Need and Demand for Inpatient Services, sponsored by the Bureau of Health Planning and Resources Development, U.S. Department of Health, Education, and Welfare, February 3-5, 1975), p. 1.

17. Ibid., p. 19.

18. Brown, op. cit., p. 36.

19. Charles G. Richie, "A Health Care Decision System" (Paper presented at the Symposium on Methods for Determining and Projecting Need and Demand for Acute Inpatient Services, sponsored by the Bureau of Health Planning and Resources Development, U.S. Department of Health, Education, and Welfare, February 3-5), 1975, p. 1.

20. Ibid., p. 23.

21. Bureau of Health Planning and Resources Development, "Methodological Approaches for Determining Health Manpower Supply and Requirements," in *Practical Planning Manual*, vol. II (Rockville, Md.: Department of Health, Education, and Welfare, 1976), HRA 76-14512, p. 36.

22. Mara Minerva Melum, *Assessing the Need for Hospital Beds: A Review of Current Criteria* (Minneapolis: Interstudy, 1975), p. 8.

23. Paul M. Press, "A Community Health Systems Analysis Method for Estimating the Need for Acute Inpatient Facilities" (Paper presented at the Symposium on Methods for Determining and Projecting Need and Demand for Acute Inpatient Services, sponsored by the Bureau of Health Planning and Resources Development, U.S. Department of Health, Education, and Welfare, February 3-5, 1975), p. 1.

24. Bureau of Health Planning and Resources Development, op. cit., p. 39.

25. American Hospital Association, *The Practice of Planning in Health Care Institutions* (Chicago: American Hospital Association, 1973), p. 8.

26. Melum, op. cit., p. 50.

27. A. Gittelsohn and J. E. Wennberg, "Health Care Delivery in Maine I: Pattern of Use of Common Surgical Procedures," *Journal of the Maine Medical Association* 66 (May 1975): 126.

28. Ibid., p. 149.

Chapter 6

Planning and Public Accountability

Clayton Medeiros

This chapter was written by Clayton Medeiros in his private capacity. No official support or endorsement by the Public Health Service Region II is intended or should be inferred.

Power always thinks it has a great soul and vast views beyond the comprehension of the weak and that it is doing God's service when it is violating all his laws.

John Adams

Basically our problem is still the central issue of the debate in the federalist papers as to whether or not the people can be trusted.

Saul Alinsky

Planning and accountability are terms about which there is little agreement, and this chapter does not propose to suggest meanings that will be either appropriate or acceptable to everyone. Further, no attempt is being made to treat the terms comprehensively, but only to present a view of their use as they are linked in the author's perspective to health planning in general and specifically in the context of the National Health Planning and Resources Development Act, PL 93-641.

In this discussion, an assumption is made that planning is intervention and that this position is reflected in PL 93-641. To the extent that planning does more than produce documents for balancing library stacks and becomes involved in implementation and resource management and allocation, there is an a priori need for accountability, and no justification will be posed.

The National Health Planning and Resources Development Act (NHPRD) takes an interventionist position in relation to the health system. In the "Findings and Purpose" Section 2(b) it states, "In recognition of the magnitude of the problems described in subsection (a) and the urgency placed on their solution, it is the purpose of this Act to facilitate the development of recommendations for a national health policy, to augment areawide and state planning for health services, manpower, and facilities, and to authorize financial assistance for the development of resources to further that policy." Although it can be questioned whether or not Congress has provided the necessary financial support to fulfill this intention, there is additional interventionist rhetoric.

Priorities are set ranging from emphasis on primary care for the medically underserved to training physicians assistants and developing effective health education methods in Section 1502. More specifically, regional health systems agencies (HSAs) are established in Section 1513 "for the purpose of-

1. improving the health of residents of a health service area,

2. increasing the accessibility (including overcoming geographic, architectural, and transportation barriers), acceptability, continuity and quality of the health services provided them,

3. restraining increases in the cost of providing the health services, and

4. preventing unnecessary duplication of health resources. . . ." The act goes on to require various reviews and establishes a review relationship with the federal government [Section 1513(e)(1)(A)] and state government [Section 1513(f)].

There is no requirement here that there be no ". . . interference with existing patterns of private professional practice of medicine, dentistry, and related healing arts" as was the case in 1966 in the preamble to PL 89-749 that established comprehensive health planning agencies. Congress, among others, is saying that we have not effectively interfered and the health system is in chaos; it is time to interfere. Congress is not pointing the finger; it is simply assessing a situation and recommending a general direction for action. That the direction for action includes a strong emphasis on planning is in keeping with national initiatives in economic, land use, and other types of planning.

PL 93-641 is unique in the comprehensiveness with which it approaches planning for health and with the opportunities that it provides to link planning and regulatory activities. In the United States, regulation tends to be heavily procedural, but not related to long range planning. When planning is a factor, it is usually the data and plans of the regulated that have provided the basis for decisions. Accountability occurs, if at all, at the decisionmaking point and not during the planning process. Such procedural accountability has great limitations, and the dependence on those regulated for information as well as for plans brings the entire effort into question.

Under the NHPRD Act, the possibilities for linking planning and regulation are inherent. The health systems plans and state health plans can be (they are not required to be) related directly to CON decisions at the state level. Such a relationship can add to procedural accountability through publicly accessible planning processes and documents that set a framework and a baseline for decisionmaking.

The following discussion is directly related to nongovernmental, not-for-profit HSAs and what is expected of health providers as they plan. The implications for states and others will be addressed. However, the HSA and its constituencies of providers, public officials, and consumers will be the focus. Although many states in conjunction with their HSAs will develop common formats, methods, and taxonomies for planning, implementation tends to be at the local level. Thus, the point of accountability also tends to be local.

Although PL 93-641 does not directly address institutional planning, there is a clear implication that institutions as they plan for the short as well as the long run should look to Health Systems Plans and State Health Plans for guidance. The basic planning functions, processes, and relations to regulation mentioned in this chapter apply with equal strength to institutional as well as HSA planning. At the institutional level, there are pressures to be open in process and clear about assumptions as services are expanded or added. The data about institutions that HSAs collect will be accessible to the public, and the institution must be prepared to work in the participatory arena. In addition, some states such as New Jersey and Washington have moved to require institutional planning that will assist in regional and state planning efforts as well as in regulation activities under CON.

There are links between institutional and HSA planning methodologically as well as environmentally. Institutions and the HSAs must deal with the state government, and it is state government that constitutionally is responsible for regulation under its police powers with regard to public health and safety. It is the state that will choose functionally to integrate planning and regulation as allowed and encouraged under PL 93-641. Not only can planning and capital expenditures and services controls be regulated, but they can be further supported by rate regulation activities. Such a tripartite effort appears to offer a solid basis for providing direction to the future development of the health system and its institutions. This is not mythic; Maryland, New York, New Jersey, Massachusetts, Rhode Island, Washington, and Wisconsin, among others, have moved or are moving in this direction.

ACCOUNTABILITY: WHAT IT MEANS

Since there is much disagreement over the term accountability, some effort will be made to provide a framework for the discussion beginning with some basic definitions. Webster defines *accountable* as "subject to giving an account; answerable (every sane man in answerable to his conscience for his behavior). . . . Capable of being accounted for; explainable. . ." He also defines *account* as "a record of debit and credit entries chronologically posted to a ledger page . . . a statement of exposition of underlying or explanatory reasons, causes, grounds or motives" and "to calculate the numerical quantity of . . ."[1] To account for something is to be answerable and responsible for it. At a general level the simple counting of an amount received is used to provide the buyer with accountability from the seller. This is an audit function and, "Without audit, no accountability, without accountability no control, where is the seat of power?"[2]

As Normanton points out, audit can be used to assure that governmental agencies are operating within the parameters set by some basic principles:

   . . . not to spend money for illegal or unauthorized purposes

   . . . observe common regulations for accounting and financial procedure

   . . . keep accounts correctly and honestly

   . . . comply with the budget and spend within its limits.[3]

He goes on to note:

   . . . financial control passes through a planning phase before the time of payment and through an accountability phase thereafter. The planning phase, during which the nature of future transactions is decided, sets the framework for accountability. After payment there will be a general investigation and a comparison of actual performance with the planned framework; this is the accountability phase. In a well-ordered and modern system the findings of the second phase contribute substantially towards the pattern of future planning.[4]

Planning requires accountability, and accountability requires planning. The plan, as stated above, "sets the framework for accountability," and accountability or the lack of it provides an input into future iterations of the plan. If the plan proposes some quantifiable amount of primary care services in the future, it provides a basis for determining whether or not that amount was actually developed. Thus the plan provides for simple accounting, but it also brings its own techniques and proposals as well as thoroughness into question if they do not reflect reality. A decision based on an articulated plan with a documented procedure for its development becomes public by the very means of the derivation of that decision and its conformance or lack of conformance with the plan.

The accountability described by Webster and of concern to Normanton is difficult to identify in the health system. The government can count the numbers and types of surgical procedures that it receives for its money as a third party payor, but it has great difficulty determining the quality of those operations. The patient must also live with the long term effects of the procedures and yet may not be aware of what those effects could be. Rarely, as Normanton observes, can the patient conduct "a general investigation and a comparison of actual performance with the planned framework," and equally rare is a thorough explanation of assumptions and technical alternatives provided to the patient.

The concerns of patients, providers, and planners are at best, difficult to articulate comprehensively and to differentiate meaningfully. The patients want good health care to assure that they get better as rapidly as possible with minimal cost and discomfort. The providers wish to deliver highest quality services that are up to date and sanctioned by colleagues. The planners want an effective and efficient system for the least possible cost. Each of these participants in the health system will have his own sense of what accountability is and is not. Who is accountable to whom on what basis becomes a focus of debate and tension. The articulation of roles and responsibilities in working within the present health boundaries and in molding the basis for determining future boundaries is important. The plan does tend to move us from the present usually ad hoc decisionmaking environment to a position where decisions at least consider the framework of a community-based plan. Does this decision on the part of this group of actors appear logical in light of what our plan articulates for our health system in five years?

The subject at hand is health and the accounting to be made is unique. In discussing audit Normanton concludes that there is a need to go beyond accounting to social responsibility where cost must be evaluated outside the columns of the ledger. Planning and health under PL 93-641 are linked at least to procedural accountability by virtue of the act, as pointed out above. They are additionally bound by the nature of the health system and processes that planners are using to pursue future directions in that system. Just as financial feasibility of an institutional project must be examined in the light of the health service area's capacity to support that project, so is financial audit being expanded to include social audit. The long range effects of a particular capital investment must be considered too, rather than just the mere ability to make the investment. Did the project follow the basic rules of accounting and did it serve the people it was supposed to serve in the way intended?

At a general level, accountability attempts to place responsibility. To turn again to Webster, "Responsible: likely to be called upon to answer . . . answerable as the primary cause, motive or agent whether of evil or good; creditable or chargeable with the result."[5] The placement of responsibility is the most difficult aspect of achieving accountability, particularly in the amorphousness of the health system and the planning field where responsibilities tend to be softly defined and widely diffused. Nonetheless, some significant efforts toward accountability can be made through the health planning process and the plan document itself.

The plan does provide a means for assessing as well as delegating responsibility to groups within the system. If there is documentation that there are too many medical surgical beds in a community and insufficient ambulatory services, the actors in the future development of services have a responsibility to deemphasize medical-surgical beds and to emphasize ambulatory services. The plan is a guide to future directions and is a basis for evaluating proposed additions to or changes in the delivery pattern. If an exception to the plan is made, the reasons for variance require specification whether they are technical, political, or some mixture of the two. The plan provides notice to providers and public officials that community need will be the basis for regulating new developments.

ACCOUNTABILITY: WHY?

The health system is unique.

> The health field, as presently constituted, lacks the economic incentives or accountability of the market place and its discipline of consumer choice. Health care exists in a 'no-man's-land' where the ultimate buyer, the patient, does not make the decisions as to whether or not to purchase services, nor does he have the opportunity to influence the purchasing power of his health care dollar by having available alternatives. The patient is therefore seeking avenues of influence over the organization and function of the health care system.[6]

The patients are not alone in their search; providers, government, and third party payors, among others, are all seeking influence. PL 93-641 is one aspect of the effort to influence the health system through planning, regulation, and participation. The public nature of the system and its potential effect on the very lives of those who use it have led to its regulation. One aspect of this view has been expressed by the utilities legal expert A.J.G. Priest:

> Why should regulation of the health care industry be analogous to the fixing of public utility rates and practices? Basically, because the business of health care is deeply and intimately affected with a public interest, because hospitals and like institutions have the power of exploitation in some measure even though it is not frequently exercised; and because such instrumentalities carry on what is in some respects a natural monopoly. And, as has long been recognized as a matter of economies as well as law, when necessity of life is provided by a monopoly or quasi-monopoly, effective regulation of that enterprise is required to protect the public interest . .."[7]

Although the monopolistic and other type qualities that the above quotes claim the health system is imbued with are disputable, the basic fact that it is imbued with the public interest is unquestionable.

The health system and its components have been treated uniquely. Much of the system is in the not-for-profit private sector, dedicated to serving a social purpose. The following has been said of voluntary hospitals, but it applies equally well to the health system generally.

> . . . they have been treated with great consideration by the authorities and have usually received the benefit of every legal doubt—from the days when injured patients were prohibited from collecting damages for the negligence of hospital employees. . . to the leaning over backward of the Public Health Service and Social Security Administration in the effort to certify as many hospitals as possible for medicare.
>
> The reason for this legal tolerance and administrative gentleness are complex and have to do with such varied factors as the persistent medical mystique, the inherent reluctance of laymen to interfere with matters even remotely connected with the practice of medicine, the feeling that hospitals are, by and large, run by dedicated people who are doing the best they can under very difficult circumstances, the absence of overt profit-making . . . .[8]

The inherent assumption of the legitimacy of charitable institutions generally and the human services professions specifically in their various actions is no longer simply accepted. The key to this shift in attitude has tended to be the rapid inflation that has taken place since the creation of Medicaid and Medicare as well as the more general professional demystifications of the sixties.

In recent public administration literature, the hospital has tended to be placed in what is called the third sector. The third sector is differentiated from the public and private sectors in that it is made up of organizations such as museums, philanthropic foundations, voluntary hospitals, etc. to perform functions not otherwise served. In some instances they are a meeting of public and private interests such as PSROs or HSAs. These latter organizations are the result of what Etzioni calls "convergent trends." He states that " 'convergent' trends in our post industrial society . . . lead to cooperative efforts at solving problems among all sectors (public, private and third) of society." These organizations are also referred to as "transorganizations" or "multiorganizational conjoins" because they are caught in a " 'web of tensions' which blurs the traditional distinctions between public and private organizations."[9]

The hospital, various forms of group practice, many physicians, planning organizations, and health regulatory bodies are functioning in the third sector environment. Their roles, responsibilities, and relationships place them there. They are closely tied to public and private arenas with much of the traditional differentiation between those arenas obscured. Regulation, payment, and planning in health all emanate from an amalgam of governmental and private sources of authority that are inextricably linked. Government's role in paying for health care is rapidly increasing directly and indirectly. Regulation comes in the payment system from government directly through Medicaid and Medicare and from a combining of direct and indirect methods through other third party payors such as Blue Cross or private insurors (insurance itself being regulated). If laissez-faire was ever alive in the health care delivery system, it is now quite ill, if not dead. The public hand is clearly visible.

This is not to say that the public hand is all-powerful. It is not. The third sector is not dominated by government; rather it sits between governmental and private functions and mixes the two. Private physicians and private hospitals remain private; however, they must be ever cognizant of their public responsibilities, many of which are going to be increasingly regulated and planned for.

McGill and Wooten have differentiated the third sector management issues from the traditional Weberian management concerns. A few comparisons will give the flavor in a loose interpretation of their analysis.

THIRD SECTOR	WEBERIAN
• goals are ambiguous, stated as directions	• goals are well defined and the time framed
• goals are in flux before and after action and are externally influenced	• goals generate from a rational means/ends process and are internally derived
• goals are informal and substantive with conflict between operations and stated goals	• goals are formal and functional with little operational conflict over goals and operations
• the institution's structure is adaptive with change ever present in a dialectic between the organization and the environment	• the structure is resistant to change, hierarchical and institutionally protective.[10]

The characteristics of the third sector are inherent in most aspects of the health system and its institutions. Public and private roles are blurred with the government taking on much of the financial burden thus under-cutting traditional charity concepts. As stated above, physicians, hospitals, and group practices, among others, along with the organizations that plan and regulate for and with them in many instances fall into the third sector. Not-for-profit HSAs and state level voluntary health councils are also included. If one agrees with this placement of many health agencies and institutions in the third sector, there are some characteristics of accountability that must be considered in relation to health planning. For example, planning tends to be based on a rational and systematic view of the world that for purposes here can be characterized as Weberian. Yet, HSAs operate in a third sector context that requires flexibility, adaptation, and constant information exchange.

As stated earlier, planning is intervention under PL 93-641, and, to the extent that planning agencies intervene, the schizoid tendency of rational/institutional integrity versus working in an open-ended health system will be apparent and will require careful monitoring. The focus of this monitoring will be participatory and geared to the agency's products such as plans and to its functions, including reviews and recommendations for regulatory purposes. Such monitoring must go well beyond simple legal requirements; it must be grounded in community needs and demands and in informal as well as formal roles and responsibilities.

The qualities of the third sector provide creative as well as limiting opportunities in planning and accountability. The HSA, for example, is in a position to play the convenor, facilitator, and mediator between the public and private sectors. Its board of directors consists of public, private, and third sector representatives, and its roles and responsibilities cut across all three sectors. For example, under Section 1513(e) of the act, the HSA has review and approval authority over certain federally funded programs. Its decision to disapprove can be overturned by the Secretary of HEW. This is a governmental, regulatory function.

The basis for the HSA's review or approval decision includes, among other requirements under Section 1532, consideration of its Health Systems Plan. The act of making a decision is in the public sector and governmental, the HSA is in the private sector as a not-for-profit corporation, and the health systems plan is between the two sectors. The plan must be considered in the governmental decision by the private organization, but the plan is not legally binding in and of itself. The plan is a series of recommendations—albeit quite specific ones—that bridge private, public, and third sector functions. Amidst this confusion, there are opportunities to move beyond the highly restrictive hierarchical bureaucracy and its attendant legal powers to a more flexible structure with significant legal authority tempered by participation and openness.

The administrator of health institutions operates in the midst of the third sector with the possible exception of proprietary organizations. The administrator has similar responsibilities to the staff of the HSA in terms of planning and managing under the overall direction of a board of trustees or directors. Just as the health planner must relate to practitioners in the development of criteria and standards for planning, so must the administrator relate to chiefs of services with their individual concerns and viewpoints. The managers in the health field, be they planners or administrators, must operate in the framework of the third sector environment. They also must be knowledgeable about regulation and its implications for capital expenditures and rates and service expansions or contractions. They are the technocrats of the health system and will increasingly stand between the users and the providers of services. Their functions must be specified so that they remain accountable. The arcane jargon of systems planning and systems management must not be allowed totally to mystify those who use and provide the services. The technocrats should not replace the physician as the shaman of health.

PLANNING TECHNIQUE: RELATION TO ACCOUNTABILITY

The previous sections of this chapter have presented a view of the need for and the environment of planning and accountability in the health system. Planning and regulation are here to stay regardless of the survival of PL 93-641. The growth and costs of health services and the dependence of the user on the provider's judgement have brought about the need for regulation and planning. State and local planning activities, whether under the auspices of the present act or some other congressional initiative, are necessary. The direct relationship of planning activities to regulation also has the ring of conventional wisdom as well as the backing of the state government's inherent constitutional authority to regulate for purposes of public health and safety.

PL 93-641 is not the panacea for planning, regulation, or accountability. It follows the conventional wisdom belatedly and fails to require links among planning, rate regulation, and CON. Rate regulation tests in six states, ten years after Medicaid and Medicare, is patently absurd. In addition, it is left to the states to provide the link between health systems plans, state plans, and CON. In a review of 20 states and 36 planning areas, Lewin and Associates, Inc. concluded that CON or capital expenditures and services (CES) controls "and rate regulation are essential and complementary."

> Rate Review, without CES planning and regulation, runs the risk of causing a long-term deterioration in the capital assets of the health care system as a result of short term "marginal cost" decisions. At the same time, even the best existing CES controls will tend to optimize health care supply around identified needs and technological developments and, by not weighing 'marginal cost' considerations, will tend to price health care beyond our means. In order for federal policy aims in health to be met, it is imperative that DHEW support a balanced health regulatory strategy.[11]

Neither Congress nor HEW has a strategy, except moderately, to encourage states in that direction.

There is a need to link CES controls, planning, and rate regulation because one element cannot be effective without the other if a rational approach is to be taken. As Lewin makes clear, short term decisions based solely on rate considerations could cause a hospital's capital base to deteriorate. Consideration must be given to depreciation factors and how capital expenditures are funded and the long range institutional plans and their impact on the hospital's rates in five or more years. The hospital's plan for long range development is viewed in the context of the regional Health Systems Plan and its proposals for the development of facilities and services. At the same time, the planner or the consumer, in attempting to satisfy needs generally or in relation to new technologies, must consider the impact on rates now and over time. A given technical innovation will cause reconsideration of:

- Health Systems Plan services and facilities aspects
- Long range and short range institutional plans
- Present, proposed, and future rates to accommodate the innovations

The short range effort to fulfill a community need through a technique such as computerized tomography may create a drastic increase in the long range rate of paying for that service as well as other services to which that service relates.

Just as no part of the health system is totally unrelated to other parts, so is no part of the planning and regulatory effort totally unrelated to the other. A long range plan can provide a framework for institutional planning and rate regulation; capital expenditures and services controls can provide support for the planning goals. Thus, an institution that emphasizes ambulatory services in keeping with a Health Systems Plan should be supported and not penalized through a rate-setting authority.

Marginal costs, which are the additional costs of producing another unit of output, are critical both to the institution and the planner, both of whom want effective services. This is particularly true in bed need studies where marginal costs are difficult to determine and average costs are commonly used. If you are producing five units of service for $100, the average cost is $20. The marginal cost of producing one more unit may not be $20, because many costs have already been met in producing the first five units. One more unit might actually decrease the average cost of all units. This is a simplified example, but it does speak to Lewin's findings.

Again, the link between the institutional administrator and the planner is apparent. Both must be concerned with the capacity and costs of the present system, the projected structure and costs of the future system, and the methods for assuring that the developments from now into the future are effective. Program plans and long range plans must be carefully evaluated as to their impact and relevance to future goals. The commonality of cost concerns is most apparent as we move toward what many are predicting will be a decade of scarce resources.

In the following discussion, the term planning is used generally as it is described in PL 93-641, that is, long range, goal-oriented systems planning. Hyman has described this approach,[12] and it is generally the systematic, rational development of long range goals based on analysis of aspects of the present health system, forecasting a future system, establishing objectives, positing alternative programs, implementing, and beginning again. This is somewhat simplified, and detailed discussions abound with Hyman. His bibliography is an excellent resource as are guidance materials from the Bureau of Health Planning and Resources Development, available through the National Health Planning Information Center.[13]

Planning techniques can be used to clarify situations and to provide and evaluate alternative solutions to problems. When used this way, the assumptions behind the techniques, the clarifications, the evaluations, and the alternatives are explicitly stated. However, planning techniques can also be used to confuse situations and limit consideration and evaluation of alternatives. When used this way, assumptions are simply obfuscations and technical jargon accompanied by numerous equations in which supposed professionalism predominates. To use a basic example, it is common practice among discussants to use averages to make a point, and averages can be quite impressive. The average life span of a given group of males might be 70 years. The average is determined by summing all of the ages of the group members and dividing by the total number of members. This is an eminently reasonable way to do things as long as one has some idea of how many persons of what types were in the group. A study done in a community of retirees would be vastly different from a study done in a college community. As stated above, assumptions must be explicit. A key to accountability lies in the techniques of planning, the explication of assumptions, and the publicness of the plan development process. Discussions of health have often suffered at the hands of supporters of sacred cows, and health planning is no different. Please note that the following discussion is not meant to be inclusive, nor is it meant to belittle planning. It is simply an attempt to provide one way of looking at accountability in the planning process envisioned in PL 93-641.

Hyman notes that "while a lack of planning theory may exist, much is available on the planning process, planning models and definitions."[14] We now have federal definitions of much health planning terminology as one example. The lack of an accepted theoretical base, however, leads the planning field to be far more concerned with means than it is with ends. If one accepts this position, the planner may be responsible for developing a rational methodology for achieving what may or may not be a rational, or, for that matter, a moral end. Those who are not responsible for the determination of ends will many times deny responsibility for the means used to achieve them.

Planners use techniques and methods, and Webster again provides a perspective: "Technique: the way in which technical details are treated;

as; the manner in which a creative artist uses the technical elements of his art to express himself." Note that the elements, not the end product, are the focus. Webster's definition of method offers further insight: "A procedure or process for attaining an objective; a systematic procedure, technique or set of rules employed in philosophical inquiry; a particular approach to problems of truth or knowledge."[15] It is the approach to truth or knowledge, but the method or technique is not *The Truth*. A series of techniques may be used to document, for example, that in the borough of Manhattan in New York City there is an overabundance of acute care hospital beds and physicians—particularly specialists. One could conclude that, therefore, the inhabitants of Manhattan must be healthy. But the techniques that identify the availability of services do not have any direct relationship to people's health. For that matter, neither do the services. If services are not accessible and affordable, they are useless.

Many planners have traditionally taken the posture that they simply provide the decision-maker with alternatives. This chapter disavows that posture as unreasonable because planning techniques for identifying need or proposing future alternative programs are not neutral, but judgmental. Many decision-makers can be misled because the underlying basis for data or methods has not been explained to them. The position of this paper is:

1. planning is intervention, and

2. the very techniques used to define and resolve a problem may provide the basis for an implicit solution.

In a HSA the board is primarily accountable as the decision-maker, but the planners are an important element of the agency's accountability even though their position is secondary. This applies to institutional administrators as well.

Planning is only one aspect of accountability and decisionmaking. As Brown et al. point out, "The planning techniques and methods are not final output goods that can be evaluated in their own right, and thus assume their own integrity. If this were true, then the health system would be forced to adapt to a preconceived or idealistic 'planning approach' instead of responding to the demands for services that are placed upon it."[16] The techniques are not self-sufficient, they are tools. "If technical planning decisions are incorporated into the planning function as an input to negotiated solution, they are considered as a positive influence that will result in a more acceptable solution."[17]

Planning is strongly grounded in measurement and in projecting measurement into the future. Planning is also grounded in value judgments, and its normative quality should be foremost in the minds of those who wish to keep it accountable. The techniques and the measurements provide a baseline of information with which a decision can be made. They are not and should not be the decision, and they provide only one part of the context for the normative decision, which also considers cultural, social, and other factors not particularly subject to measurement.

Gordon is cited as saying:

> There are some important caveats about forecasting the future that must be noted. First, there is no way to state what the future will be. Regardless of the sophistication of the methods, all rely on judgements, not fact.
>
> Second, there will always be blind spots in forecasts. If we try to guess what will happen in the future, we are likely to omit events for which there will be no existing [theory]... and events based on whim, chance and unexpected coincidence.[18]

In the preceding chapter, Crane cites five methods for assessing bed needs, including regression formulas, and stochastic methods, among others. Regression basically incorporates a series of independent variables into an equation to extrapolate future values of a dependent variable. There are many problems, including the problem of numerous variables not being as quantifiable as necessary for purposes of the analysis. Hill-Burton formulas have well-known limitations, particularly the assumption of the current utilization rate remaining constant over time and the inability to address effectively service types and locations. Stochastic models tend to be institutionally rather than regionally applicable. All of the above issues are clearly and concisely discussed by Brown et al.[19] They specify some propositions with regard to assessing bed need, two of which are noted that directly relate to accountability:

> ... Since the bed need assessment techniques will not specify the types of service to be offered in a region, locality, or hospital, the exchange of information between planners and providers is critical so that a balance between technical feasibility and social desirability may be met. 4. The results of bed need assessment techniques are primarily technically and economically rational solutions which tend to create an impetus for a political rationality to implement these solutions. The techniques, however, being technically oriented, cannot account for the divergence of a technical or economic solution with other politically optimal solutions.[20]

In summation, the social and political must be weighed with the technical. The values of the community are the leaven for the bread of planning technique. The planning technique is accountable to the extent that its assumptions are explicit. Secondarily, the assumptions are far easier to clarify to a board or review committee than the techniques themselves. Such clarification appropriately strengthens the normative hand of the decision-maker, alleviates the inclination to turn board members into working technicians, and provides accountability for providers as well as for consumers. Many times, both parties can be equally bowled over by the systems jargon of the planner. Using assumptions as a technical starting point and realizing the value-laden quality of the final judgement provide a basis for making the planners accountable to:

- those being planned for and with
- the decision-maker
- the community at large
- themselves

The techniques for manipulating formulas or fitting various curves in regression are not in and of themselves important to board members or committee members. The committee should, however, understand the assumptions that underlie the use of a curve. A linear projection of data from five past years into five future years keyed only to population growth results in the past's being the sole basis for judging the future. Utilization patterns in pediatrics, for example, assume that the past utilization will be the future utilization modified for population. Projections other than linear have their own package of assumptions that require specification, aside from the technical problems involved in forecasting population growth or decline in the first place. The decision-makers need to know and can understand the assumptions without necessarily thoroughly understanding the techniques themselves.

Health planning and its associated techniques are recent additions to both the planning and health fields. However, we have had a long history of analysis in which practitioners and academics have placed special emphasis on using basic techniques to point out possible solutions to identified problems. Yet our present level of knowledge is not as great as some would like it to be; however, it is not as limited as some would lead us to believe.

We are not using on a national basis many of the techniques available to us, as Brown points out. PL 93-641 provides an opportunity to identify for practitioners the present state of the profession and to focus on dissemination of that state far and wide, including documentation of limitations. This is not to demote the benefits of research into new methods; it is simply the statement of a need to use effectively what now exists. (The details of some planning methods are discussed in Chapter five.) The fact that so few states have effective planning and regulatory programs speaks to the failure of techniques to be widely disseminated and applied. Of course, resource limitations are also a factor.

THE PLAN AS ACCOUNTABILITY

In any system there is a tendency to lose sight of goals in the face of day-to-day activities. This is particularly true of third sector, convergent organizations. The position taken in this discussion is that health systems organizations, be they hospitals or HSAs, must tread a line between the Weberian, hierarchical view and the existential, third sector view. In order to assure accountability, goals and plans are necessary, but to be responsive to social needs and demands, flexibility is essential.

To the extent that a publicly derived plan articulates and specifies goals and objectives (quantifiably and time framed where possible), it assists in preserving them as the focus of resources and actions. They do not get lost in the hustle and bustle of brushfires and instant decisions as opposed to long range policy development. If nothing else, under PL 93-641, they are annually reviewed.

For all of its 52 pages, as noted above, the National Health Planning and Resource Development Act provides a great deal of process, but calls for very little accountability. Plans, reviews, data analysis, meetings, etc., will be undertaken and appropriate documents for next year's federal grant generated, but it could all be done with a modicum of responsibility at anything greater than a superficial level.

Process does provide a level of accountability, and due process will be strongly evident in review and regulation. The requirements for openness will also assist, since records and documents of all kinds are public in the HSA. Section 1532 (b) provides an excellent example of procedural as opposed to substantive requirements:

(b) Each health systems agency and State Agency shall include in the procedures required by subsection (a) at least the following:

1. Written notification to affected persons of the beginning of a review.

2. Schedules for reviews which provide that no review shall, to the extent practicable, take longer than ninety days from the date the notification described in paragraph (1) is made.

3. Provision for persons subject to a review to submit to the agency or State Agency (in such form and manner as the agency or State Agency shall prescribe and publish) such information as the agency or State Agency may require concerning the subject of such review).

4. Submission of applications (subject to review by a health systems agency or a State Agency) made under this Act or other provisions of law for Federal financial assistance for health services to the health systems agency or State Agency at such time and in such manner as it may require.

5. Submission of periodic reports by providers of health services and other persons subject to agency or State Agency review respecting the development of proposals subject to review.

6. Provision for written findings which state the basis for any final decision or recommendation made by the agency or State Agency.

7. Notification of providers of health services and other persons subject to agency or State Agency review of the status of the agency or State Agency review of the health services or proposals subject to review, findings made in the course of such review, and other appropriate information respecting such review.

8. Provision for public hearings in the course of agency or State Agency review if requested by persons directly affected by the review; and provision for public hearings, for good cause shown respecting agency and State Agency decisions.

9. Preparation and publication of regular reports by the agency and State Agency of the reviews being conducted (including a statement concerning the status of each such review) and of the reviews completed by the agency and State Agency (including a general statement of the findings and decisions made in the course of such reviews) since the publication of the last such report.

10. Access by the general public to all applications reviewed by the agency and State Agency and to all other written materials pertinent to any agency or State Agency review.

As Boyer and Weiner note, there are many aspects to accountability: public, post-audit, pre-audit, products, projects, institutional, process, fiscal, social, political, public, etc. It is a massive subject. Boyer and Weiner share the author's view that in addition to public accountability, there is participatory accountability.[21] PL 93-641 potentially provides for accountability through its emphasis on open, public actions and participation in the planning and other type activities of HSAs.

Under PL 93-641, the not-for-profit HSA is the fount of accountability and fits in with the third sector schema. It represents a convergence of public and private roles in review and comment/recommendation or approval (subject to overturn on appeal to higher authority). It also provides an opportunity to differentiate the de jure and de facto aspects of accountability.

The term de jure is defined in Webster's as "by right: of right by a lawful title." The term de facto is defined as "actually; in fact; in reality; exercising the powers and demanding the privileges of a regularly and legally constituted authority often with a color of right." The most common use of these terms is in giving recognition to governments formed by revolution or coup. De jure recognition of a government is recognition by right in law. De facto recognition means that one is recognized as actually controlling the government, but is not recognized by right in law. To oversimplify the example a bit further, it is a question of law versus reality; de jure the speed limit is 55 miles per hour, but de facto one is rarely stopped for doing 60 miles per hour.

PL 93-641 has a great deal of de jure accountability in the form of detailed procedural requirements for being designated and receiving a grant. The underlying procedures, however, are unclear, and de facto accountability will depend on the level and intensity of participation in each area. The HSA is to make reports as required, to provide for fiscal controls and accounting procedures, and to provide audit access to the Secretary under Section 1512(b)(6). This is traditional accountability and required of all federal grantees. This will not provide functional information with regard to planning.

Other requirements are outlined for board selection and are quite specific with regard to providers, indirect providers, consumers and public officials. The enumeration, however, stops there and does not provide guidance for the selection of specific representatives, nor does it assure that a "good" process will be used. There are numerous de jure requirements and definitions, but "good" process will occur based as much on de facto considerations such as the informal relationships within a community among the leaders of business, medicine, community action and religious groups and the compromises made before, during, and after formal meetings.

Under the de jure requirements, it is quite possible that some HSAs will be as self-perpetuating as some CHPs, hospitals, and other health institutions have been in selecting their boards of directors or boards of trustees. Of course, if the act and its regulations were any more specific, there would be much hue and cry about federal interference, and appropriately so. Federal law can provide only a basis or a framework that makes responsibility and accountability possible; it cannot directly provide such responsibility and accountability.

Direct participation is the only means to assure that what one wants to accomplish is going forward. Direct does not simply mean participation on the board; many committees for review and planning have more policy impact than the board. Also, the public quality of the agency's records provides for external and internal monitoring. It could be said that so much monitoring might go on that little planning will take place. Again, the general requirements placed on HSAs for plans and reviews make this unlikely. However, the same issue noted with regard to board structure is present here as well. HSAs must plan, but there will be great difficulty in judging the quality of what they do. The requirements for final designation of an HSA allow for a period of 12 or 24 months. To be finally designated, an agency must have an acceptable Health Systems Plan. If a 12-month final designation is wanted, the planning process will be quite rushed. The rush will continue as in future years additional federal, congressional, and state requirements continue to put pressure on HSAs to produce ever better plans.

De jure and de facto accountability are essential to the functions of an HSA. Direct participation on boards and committees assists in assuring accountability at the level of day-to-day actions and tends to operate in the de jure world of law and regulatory requirements. To further assure that those requirements are fulfilled, informal as well as formal monitoring must take place—formal monitoring through reports on actions and minutes of meetings and informal monitoring through interest groups impacting on particular issues, through exerting political or social pressures. Overall, the open information requirements of PL 93-641 provide a formal as well as informal means of direct and indirect participation. The key is in the openness of both process and product.

A plan then provides definitions, clarifies technical assumptions, allows flexibility, and, where it is possible to quantify goals and objectives, provides accountability. The techniques are open to public inspection; the providers and the community know what to expect five or more years hence and can plan for their institutional and other needs accordingly. The publicness of the plan document and the techniques and processes used to develop it are not internal to HSA, but subject to critical evaluation by all comers. This type of plan does not dictate solutions, but provides room for alternatives to be considered so that creativity of problem solution remains possible at the institutional and community levels.

All of this may seem somewhat simple-minded, but it is one method available to achieve accountability in health planning. It aids in overcoming the problem of substituting technique for full-fledged planning and establishes a process where techniques for planning are based on assumptions that are understood and accepted by the HSAs' decision-makers.

The intensity of accountability is keyed to the purposes for which the plan is used. If the plan is to support library stacks, there is very limited accountability and participation is diffused of its meaning. If it is linked to review and regulation, required of the HSA, but not the state, (although some states, among them New York and New Jersey, intend to have such a linkage), then clearly there can be accountability. Expectations of the future health care system are explicated, and realistic institutional and community planning can take place. The plan becomes a communal decisionmaking tool. Care must be taken to assure that the plan does not become so institutionalized that its proponents defend it against any and all future changes. The plan is not to be worshipped just because it has been produced and adopted. To be meaningful and useful, it must be a flexible document.

The HSA and its plan become what Strauss, et al. have called "an invisible college" that will:

> teach the people of the communities they serve a new way of thinking and behaving about community health and health care services. This 'new way' calls for communities to invent, institute, manage, and evaluate comprehensive systems of governance and accountability for the health services industry. It calls for reallocation of resources to fit new national, state and local priorities. It calls for a move from laissez-faire to massive intervention. It calls for sensitivity to consumer perceptions and demands. It calls for these changes to be initiated in the context of a declining economy and declining resources.[22]

The need to plan appears to be perceived as more generally acceptable in the face of declining resources. Planning with an emphasis on its usefulness in intervention becomes a tool for resource allocation. The power to allocate resources requires that planning technique as well as planning process be accountable. The normative and the technical must be melded.

Planning is one tool in the process of community choice for the health system. As a writer said some time ago, "We cannot live on the human level without ideas. Upon them depends what we do. Living is nothing more or less than doing one thing instead of another."[23] And so it is with planning which attempts to provide a rationale for doing one thing rather than another. Such choice when backed by sanctions "is inseparable from power. It is natural and indeed desirable that everybody wielding any kind of power should have some sort of a plan, that is to say, that he should use power deliberately and consciously, looking some distance ahead of time."[24] Thus the determination of choice, the choosing and the doing are interwoven, and each necessitates accountability since each affects the distribution of resources.

PLAN: SUBSTANCE AND PROCESS

One of the many priorities for the content of health systems plans would appear to be primary care. Under Section 1502 of the act, the first priority is "the provision of primary care services for medically underserved populations, especially those which are located in rural or economically depressed areas." Some comprehensive health planning agencies also identified this as a priority and tried to act accordingly and, in some instances, followed the systems planning as well as process mandates of PL 93-641.

An example is the Comprehensive Health Planning Agency of Western New York (WNY). The technical and process characteristics of the WNY plan development activity deserve extensive documentation, but such documentation will not be attempted here. One small piece of the WNY plan will be used to demonstrate some aspects of the interrelationships between planning and accountability as discussed in this chapter.

WNY is a third sector organization, a not-for-profit corporation with a consumer-dominated board of directors. In addition to its CHP responsibilities, it has had authority to make CON recommendations to the state of New York. It has applied the basic techniques of long range, goal-oriented systems planning.

The board of directors of WNY considered primary care a priority and authorized a task force on primary care to develop a regional plan "that would result in guidelines that could be followed by the Planning Council, providers of care, and other interested groups so that future systems of health care could be more responsive to human need."[25] The plan was to indicate aspects that could best be addressed at regional county and subcounty levels. After much debate, a definition was heatedly and meticulously derived through an open, public task force process as follows: "Primary Care, usually ambulatory, offers an entry point and a holistic approach to personal health (patient) problems of a medical, emotional and social nature. It provides continuous and immediate care (not requiring a specialty level of expertise) with triage, coordination, referral to secondary and tertiary resources and follow up."[26]

Following this definition, the task force states, "This definition firmly establishes Primary Care as the foundation of a health care system which is vertically integrated and regionally coordinated. It is the first line of care, the entry point to a regional system, and the kind of care that most people need most of the time."[27] The primary care plan and other pieces of the WNY plan speak to eight clearly defined characteristics including:

1. Availability
2. Accessibility
3. Acceptability
4. Affordability
5. Coordination and Continuity
6. Quality
7. Accountability and Evaluation
8. Economy, Efficiency and Effectiveness[28]

In addition to being defined, each characteristic has specified objectives such as "Accessibility, objective 4. As a general rule, 30 minutes of travel time is the minimum degree of proximity acceptable for the region and in urban areas this should be less than 30 minutes by public transportation."[29]

After setting this overall, defined framework, the plan assesses each of the characteristics for the region and its subparts, including national and state-wide comparisons. Included in the assessment is the use, as a rough measure, of the Index of Medical Underservice (IMU) from the Health Maintenance Organization Act of 1973. The index is calculated using a formula:

$$IMU = V_1 + V_2 + V_3 + V_4$$
Where

V_1 = weighted value for % population below poverty level

V_2 = weighted value for % population aged 65 and over

V_3 = weighted value for infant mortality rate averaged over the four-year period 1970-1973

V_4 = weighted value for primary care physicians per 1,000 population

In using this formula, the plan and its appendices document the problems inherent in the use of indicators generally and IMUs specifically. In addition, data uses are carefully explained and all assumptions are articulated. Only then is a decision made "that areas having an IMU of less than 65.0 warrant special scrutiny."[30] Values are given for census tract, minor civil division, county, and region and are displayed on maps.

Finally, the plan makes specific recommendations—regional, local, and institutional—for each characteristic based on the findings. It concludes with "Guidelines for the Planning and Operation of Primary Health Care Services and Criteria for Establishment of Primary Care Centers."[31] The same thoroughness, intense participation, clarity of assumptions, and explanation of techniques have been applied to hospitals and long term care facilities.

Although this example is simplified, it is provided to demonstrate that the type of plan suggested by PL 93-641 is possible and has already been carried out. Such plans using available techniques can provide technical as well as procedural accountability. The WNY effort was not perfect, but it does offer one of several extant examples of accountable plan development.

PLANNING: SUBSTANCE AND REGULATION

The following example provides a basis for many of the ideas expressed in this chapter. There is an effort to provide for accountable recommendations on the part of a local health planning agency in a state with CON. There is a technical planning process in the context of committees and a board of directors. There is a normative decisionmaking process that plays out the politics of planning.

Based on a state effort to promulgate facilities plans, the Genesse Region Health Planning Council of Rochester, New York (GRC) developed an acute care (medical/surgical) plan. This plan was the product of a committee of consumers and providers that included representatives from all of the hospitals in the affected area. The methodologies used for the necessary bed studies and population estimates are specified and were agreed to by the committee and subsequently ratified by the board of directors. Thus, the basic requirement for technical assumptions to be made explicit is fulfilled.

The approved plan included a policy statement calling for a moratorium of one year on the addition of acute care beds in the affected area. The moratorium was partially based on the key finding that through 1980 there would be a need for 646 beds in the affected area and that at present there were 705 existing beds. The area was overbedded by about 60 beds. Given the facts as presented through technique, a policy conclusion was reached and a moratorium declared.

A hospital, with a clearly documented high utilization rate, applied for a CON and was reviewed by the GRC with full consideration of the findings of the plan including the following resolution:

> On the basis of the information and data it is evident that there is no apparent demonstrated need for additional medical/surgical beds in the four-county area at this time. It is also evident that, although there is excess capacity in acute-care beds in this area, this is primarily due to maldistribution among the hospitals and not as an absolute.
>
> Rather than attempt to expand medical/surgical beds anywhere in the region, it is suggested that the institutions first work toward:

> 1. Closer scrutiny of the utilization of existing beds particularly during periods of high census.
>
> 2. Changes in bed certification from those of underutilized services to those which are in excess capacity.
>
> 3. More cooperation between the Medical-surgical staff and the administration in scheduling effective surgical procedures.
>
> 4. Sharing of physicians, surgeons and specialists among hospitals.
>
> 5. Regionalization of certain Specialty Services.
>
> 6. Transfer of patients between hospitals during peak loads or emergencies.
>
> 7. Petition the State Health Department to permit greater flexibility in the use of existing beds during the periods of peak loads.

Staff arrayed data on the bed need situation, including the applicant's request for 40 additional beds within an existing structure in the various calculations of bed to population ratios. The facts of the high utilization were articulated and concurred on. The potential financial impact of a bed increase was included as follows:

While it is difficult to accurately assess the total dollar impact on the health-care system, staff has seen the methodology used by the New York State Department of Health in estimating the cost of an excess hospital bed over the 40-year life of the hospital bed. Applying that methodology to the delivery system of the area, it can be estimated that the cost of an excess bed in the system is approximately $8.8 million.

The methodology used in arriving at this estimate is as follows:

For each hospital total allowable inpatient cost (1973), adjusted patient days (bassinet days equal one-third adult days), and the number of beds were obtained and an average rate was calculated.

The weighted average was $85.74.

$ 85.74   Average weighted cost
    × 365   Days in a year
$ 31,295.10   Annual cost of operating a single bed.
      × 40   Lifespan of a bed as recognized by Blue Cross, Medicaid and several government mortgaging agencies
$1,251,804.00   Forty-year cost of a single bed on a constant cost basis
    × 7,040   Compound factor at 5% for forty years
$8,812,700.00

Additional comments on the above calculations:

- Inflates a debt service as well as operating cost. True, but it is offset by the absence of any factor for future renovations and the resulting additional debt service.

- Inflation factor represents all operating cost increases not only the purely inflationary aspects.

- Calculation requires that the bed would be staffed and ready to be used. Otherwise, the cost of an unready bed is its debt service, which would be borne by the beds in use.

The critical issue was that beds were maldistributed. Considering, articulating, and clearly arraying all of the facts, staff concluded:

As can be seen from the information presented in the staff analysis, two things appear evident:

1. There is an excess of acute-care beds . . .

2. The distribution of the existing beds among institutions and among services is less than optimal.

The . . . Plan gives full cognizance to this problem. The recommendations set forth in that plan for study, evaluation and implementation during the one-year moratorium are designed to provide ways to begin solving this problem without calling for the construction of additional acute-care beds.

While staff can be sympathetic to the problem that is sometimes experienced by patients who sometimes have to wait for a hospital bed to free up, staff cannot just write off as "bound-to-fail" the alternatives recommended in the Finger Lakes Hospital Plan.

The lifespan of a hospital bed, as recognized by Blue Cross, Medicaid and several government mortgaging agencies, is 40 years. Therefore, the solution proposed by the submission of the application would represent a very long and continuingly costly solution to a problem that might well be resolved by other means.

STAFF RECOMMENDATION
40 Medical/Surgical Beds

Disapproval on the basis of *Community Need.*
Disapproval on the basis of *Financial Impact Upon the Community.*

The sponsor has stated in previous presentations that the medical/surgical component of the application is integral to the balance of the application. Staff would, therefore, recommend disapproval of the balance of the application and encourages the sponsor to submit a new Part I application for a total ambulatory care program and any other components of a renovation and expansion program it elects to pursue. The staff recommendations were supported, the application withdrawn, and a new application for 20 beds submitted.

The same basic process occurred as outlined above. The area's institutions were part of the overall planning process and supported its technical development and the resulting policies, including the moratorium. In the specific instance at hand an exception was being requested, and the administrator of the institution was operating in the public arena of the planning agency. The de jure process of formal give and take was ongoing between the hospital administrator, the hospital's staff and board, and the planning agency's staff and committee. Each was operating openly from a technical de jure perspective, and, at the same time, a normative process of judgement was occurring around aspects of implementing policy, the moratorium and its resolution in particular.

The arena is clearly the third sector; the process is open and public at a technical and a value-judgement level; the result would be a state governmental decision to approve or disapprove based on the recommendation of a not-for-profit regional planning agency. All of the elements for planning and accountability are present.

Staff's recommendation was again negative and included a series of recommended alternatives based on the moratorium resolution such as "recertifying existing pediatric beds to medical-surgical beds because they may not meet regionalization criteria in the future and would assist the present situation." Staff carefully analyzed the utilization impact of each alternative and variations of the alternatives. They concluded:

Since population projections for the Genesee Region and all of New York State continue to be revised downward (here it is to be emphasized that the next set of population projections of the Economic Development Board of New York State is expected to show a significant reduction in the rate of projected population growth through the year 2000), and since major economic pressures to redefine the traditional methods of providing health care exist and continue to grow, health planners must exercise every possible restraint if major increases of acute-care capacity in excess of need are to be avoided.

Disapproval was recommended, but the application was nonetheless approved by the review committee.

The staff disapproval recommendation included the following discussion which is worth quoting in full (with some grammatical modification and names deleted).

Before any acute-care beds are added in the area, there should be a realistic overall assessment of the problems and needs of the area. A covert mistake which is often made when dealing with specific applications is that the review fails to take into consideration this overview of the total spectrum of problems that should be addressed. This is unfortunate because what often happens is that, while ideal solutions to problems are being ignored because of political realities of the moment, other pressures (usually economic) are building up to such a degree that all of a sudden, a larger political decision is imposed upon the community by the bureaucracies of the state or federal governments. These decisions rarely carry with them solutions which could be considered ideal for the local community.

An overall assessment of the problems and needs in the area includes the following:

1. While there is an apparent deficiency of medical/surgical beds there are excess medical/surgical beds in other parts of the area. At the same time, there are identified needs: more long-term care facilities, more inpatient and outpatient psychiatric and alcoholism facilities, and less medical/surgical beds in a number of facilities. Rather than increasing medi-

cal/surgical beds in a vacuum, the only logical answer would seem to be for the hospitals and the community to work with the planning agency on the resolution of these problems.

2. It is clear that additional medical/surgical beds are needed. At the same time, there are excess medical/surgical beds. When this problem is considered along with the increased utilization of ambulatory-care services that is coming and utilization-review requirements that are developing, then it can be seen that, when these factors are actively combined with the reduced projections in the rates at which population is expected to grow, the situation may well be aggravated.

3. At the same time that there is an overall excess of medical/surgical beds, there is a deficiency of long-term care facilities.

4. Economic pressures are such that increased use must be made of traditional home-care services and "hospital level" home-health services. As such utilization occurs, pressures on acute-care occupancy can be somewhat alleviated.

5. The Hospital Plan identified a need for increased psychiatric facilities. When one adds to this the alcoholism patients who are currently being cared for in Rochester, it becomes clear that serious consideration should be given to increasing both acute and long-term care psychiatric-bed capacity.

6. Previous studies have already identified an excess of maternity beds and obstetrical services. If we are to discuss rational alternatives to adding medical/surgical beds in a vacuum, it would appear that the time has come for the identified hospitals to help alleviate other problems by addressing the problem of excess obstetrical capacity.

7. While previous studies have not identified major problems with respect to the allocation of pediatric-bed resources in the Finger Lakes, evidence of the actions currently taking place within the New York State Department of Health (NYSDH) would suggest that this area needs additional consideration. Fiscal sanctions for occupancy rates of less than 70% have already been imposed. In addition, the state has indicated that it will require the recertification to medical/surgical of any pediatric unit of less than 16 beds.

8. As noted above, the State of New York has established a set of fiscal sanctions for penalizing institutions with low occu-

pancy. These sanctions can be imposed by service as well as for overall occupancy. Up to this time these sanctions have been little used. If the state applies them and they say they are going to, the financial penalties could be disastrous for institutions maintaining excess capacity.

Thus, it can be seen that the granting of additional medical/surgical capacity, without at the same time eliminating excess capacity where it exists, could not only aggravate the problem of medical/surgical overbedding but, when combined with the projected sanctions, could bring fiscal collapse of one or more needed institutions.

At the general policy level, the ideas were, and remain, acceptable. The plan stands. But in the particular instance, with its emotion and politics, an exception was made and the letter drafted by staff was quoted, because the reviewers' recommendation to the state cleared the air and placed the decision in its value-laden political environment:

In its review of the application the Conference also spent considerable time discussing the alternative recommendations set forth in the staff analysis. While it was in agreement that the staff analysis identified areas of change which will eventually have to be made, the members of the Conference did not feel that it was appropriate to ignore the known need for additional medical/surgical beds because of existing excesses of medical/surgical beds at other hospitals.

The Conference was satisfied that a disapproval of this application would not lead to a significant change in the medical referral patterns of the area but would, rather, merely create additional hardships for the hospital staff and the patient population which looks to the hospital staff for its medical services. Additionally, the Conference was satisfied that much of the overload that occurs because of the high occupancy rate was being referred to hospitals where the per diem costs of care approach $200 per day, rather than to other hospitals in the area.

Additionally, the Conference felt that a disapproval of the application would have the effect of being perceived as an attempt to interfere with the freedom of choice aspects that are customary to established patient selection and medical referral patterns of the health care system. The Conference did not feel that it had adequate authority to attempt to force such change.

With respect to the issue of looking to other hospitals for a voluntary decertification of beds, members of the Conference did not feel that such a voluntary decertification was likely to take place. Members of the Conference did not feel that they had the legal authority to demand such a decertification process of other area hospitals, nor did they feel that it was appropriate to continue to deny the known need for additional beds because of bed excesses at other area hospitals over which the sponsor had no control.

The example used here does not require extensive explanation. The roles of planner, institutional administrator, and the board are clear. The process was open, accountable, and technically astute. A decision was made with community values at the forefront. The administrator presented data, as did the planner. This is an example of the planning process at work. The de jure procedures were fulfilled, but de facto considerations were critical in the end. The final decision by the state of New York is pending as of this writing.

CONCLUSION

At best, accountability is difficult to achieve. Achievement appears simplest in a situation with defined boundaries, easily predictable outcomes, and straightforward issues. None of these attributes applies to the health system, and they are equally inapplicable to the planning field.

This chapter has attempted to provide a basis for consideration of some of the issues involved in health planning and accountability. It rests on assumptions that have, it is hoped, been made explicit. It posits the openness and publicness of PL 93-641 as the hope that will make health planning accountable. It suggests that participation and the eternal vigilance that accompanies meaningful involvement will assist in producing useful, accountable health plans. Finally, where resources are being allocated on a normative and a technical basis, if there is no plan, there is no accountability, and the community suffers accordingly.

Notes

1. *Webster's Third New International Dictionary*, unabridged (Springfield, Mass: G. and C. Merriam Co., 1966).
2. E.L. Normanton, "The Accountability and Audit of Governments" (New York: Frederick H. Praeger, Inc., 1966), p. vii.

3. Ibid., p. 22.

4. Ibid., p. 24.

5. Webster, op. cit.

6. William L. Kissick, in Herbert Harvey Hyman's *Health Planning: A Systematic Approach* (Germantown, Md.: Aspen Systems Corp., 1975), p. 52.

7. A. J. G. Priest, "Possible Adaptation of Public Utility Concepts in the Health Care Field," *Law and Cont. Problems* 35:840.

8. Anne R. Somers, *Hospital Regulation: The Dilemma of Public Policy* (Princeton: Princeton University, 1969), p. 143.

9. Michael E. Mcgill and Leland M. Wooton, "A Symposium: Management in the Third Sector," *Public Administration Review,* September/October 1975, p. 446.

10. Ibid., pp. 448-449.

11. Lewin and Associates, "Evaluation of the Efficiency and Effectiveness of the Section 1122 Review Process" (Washington, D.C.: U.S. Department of Health, Education, and Welfare, 1975), HRA 106-74-183, pp. 1-29.

12. Herbert H. Hyman, *Health Planning: A Systematic Approach* (Germantown, Md.: Aspen Systems Corp., 1975), p. 75.

13. National Health Planning Information Center, P.O. Box 31, Rockville, Maryland 20850.

14. Hyman, op. cit., p. 64.

15. Webster, op. cit.

16. Gordon D. Brown, Gary Candia, and Gale Gavin, *Methods for Hospital Service and Bed Need Assessment* (University Park, Pa.: Pennsylvania State University), p. 42.

17. Ibid., p. 44.

18. Ibid., p. 22.

19. Ibid., p. 38.

20. Ibid., pp. 37-38.

21. E. Gil Boyer and Joan Weiner, "Health Man Looks at Accountability and the Health Systems Agency" (Wyncote, Pa.: Communication Materials Center, 1975), p. 19.

22. Carol J. Harten, Mark A. Kempner, and Marvin D. Strauss, "Toward an Invisible College: Training of Planning Personnel for Local and State Agencies," *Public health Reports,* January/February 1976, p. 51.

23. Ortega y Gasset in E. F. Schumacher, *Small is Beautiful* (New York: Harper and Row, 1975), p. 86.

24. Ibid., pp. 234-235.

25. Comprehensive Health Planning Council of Western New York, Inc., "Primary Health Care" (Buffalo: Comprehensive Health Planning Council of Western New York, Inc., June 26, 1975), p. 1.

26. Ibid., p. 3.

27. Ibid., p. 3.

28. Ibid., p. 7.

29. Ibid., p. 8.

30. Ibid., pp. 22-23.

31. Ibid., p. 43.

32. Genesee Region Health Planning Council, Rochester, N.Y., Review Files. Remaining quotes are from various parts of that file and the Thompson application to the Genesee Council.

Chapter 7

Implications and Actions

Herbert H. Hyman

This chapter was written by Herbert H. Hyman in his private capacity. No official support or endorsement by the Health Resources Administration of HEW is intended or should be inferred.

The purpose of this final chapter is to discuss the implications for health planning posed by the various authors in this book, from the perspective of both the health planning agencies and the health providers. This chapter will also confront the issue of how providers can collaborate with the Health Systems Agency and will identify potential techniques for accomplishing a balanced working relationship.

IMPLICATIONS OF CON REGULATION

Effectiveness of CON/1122 Laws

In Harmon's chapter on the major study of CON conducted by Lewin & Associates in 1974-75, the main conclusions tended to support what others had previously contended:

1. The great majority of CON requests were approved (90% or more) with the exception of lower approval rates for new facilities.

2. The CON process was not particularly effective in its cost containment policy, as evidenced by the continued approval of projects in almost 50% of the sampled areas, despite the fact that area plans indicated that no new facilities or beds were needed.

3. The CON process was not very efficient in most areas. This was due to the relative lack of data, plans, or criteria available to the review agencies for determining need. Also, most of the CON applications themselves were poorly written and lacked specific goals, supportive data, or cost analysis.

4. Although Harmon identified a number of reasons why the CON and 1122 review processes were not effective, there was one ray of hope that

seemed to shine through the pessimism of the study. The report noted that where both prospective rate reviews and CON reviews were utilized in the same state, the cost containment policy appeared to work well.

While Harmon identified a number of reasons as to why cost containment did not work, there was one conclusion that seemed more important, namely, her contention that the federal commitment to cost containment failed to strike a responsive chord in the state or local area planning agencies. This was due to the lack of understanding as to what Section 1122 was supposed to do to bring about cost containment at the state level, and to federal policies running counter to health needs as perceived by consumers and providers at the local level. The implications of these findings are important because they strike at the heart of what is wrong with the federal cost containment policy.

First, where policy is enunciated in an ambiguous or unclear manner, it is subject to a wide range of interpretations that are used by the planning agencies, the community at large, and the health providers to achieve their own private goals. These goals are, surprisingly, more often a source of agreement than a source of conflict among the various actors. This is because those involved are generally interested in raising the quality of care in the region. There is consequently a greater tendency at the regional level to collaborate in support of such CON requests than to reject them. They mean better medical care to some, more jobs or greater prestige to others, and a sense of medical security to still others. When the ambiguity of the federal government's cost containment policy collides with specific proposals for improving medical care at the local level, the federal policy generally loses.

Second, there is no accepted standard of defining "needs." There is often confusion as to whether a definition of need (the type and level of medical services required by all members of the health service area) or a definition of demand (the resources required to provide care to those who actually use those services) should be used in developing projections for services and facilities required by the area's population. This lack of clarity causes confusion about what is really needed by which population in the community. The population that uses the medical facilities based on demand forecasts may have a different set of values and priorities about the type of medical facilities and services they require than the population who needs, but seldom uses, these same facilities. Without clear definition, each health provider and health planning agency can promote its own definition of need or demand to support its respective claim for or against a particular CON request. The competition between the providers and public officials on the opposite side is usually no contest. The provider/consumer tandem has usually prevailed and, in the process, won over the health planners to their way of thinking.

Third, the notion that one method, strategy, or process by itself is sufficient to implement a basic policy such as cost containment has been proved wrong. Fragmented as the health system is, there are, nevertheless, identifiable components of that system that impact on the cost containment policy. Among these are the individual needs of health providers and consumers for better services regardless of cost, the maintenance of the role and status of physicians in their efforts to provide the quality of care their patients demand regardless of cost, the third party payment mechanism, the process and methods for setting service rates, and the efforts of health planning agencies to improve the medical delivery system of their areas. Each one of these components, though organizationally autonomous, does impact on the efforts of the others. A strategy that does not deal with all or most of these components in a systematic and comprehensive manner cannot achieve its end, and cost containment is no exception. Harmon's analysis provides an excellent diagnosis of what is wrong and right about the federal initiative to implement its cost containment policy. However, she fails to place her own analysis of the various components in some sort of systems framework. Consequently, although she offers positive recommendations, they may not achieve the objective of cost containment because she does not consider their impact on the other components of the system. Only a systems approach to this issue can uncover the weaknesses and strengths of what is needed to achieve cost containment and to assess the impact on the system.

Fourth, the issue of cost containment will intensify rather than disappear in the future, because American society has become more conscious of how rising medical costs both increase taxes and reduce take-home pay. In the short run, the health providers can outwit and outmaneuver any law, health plan, or policy with which they are confronted in order to meet their own institution's immediate needs. However, in the long run, when the public becomes more fully aware that the increase in the cost of medical care does not necessarily purchase a commensurate amount of medical care, the resulting backlash may create demand on state and congressional legislators to enact harsher and more restrictive policies on health providers. The question is whether health providers prefer to deal with the issues involved in cost containment in a rational and thoughtful manner while they still maintain considerable influence in the health system, or be subject to a reactive, ad hoc and emotional policy that may be destructive to their own institution's and society's health needs.

Fifth, regulation as a tool to control costs is also too limited to deal with the cost containment issue. Regulation is only one phase of a system for improving the health system. Planning, resources development, use of those resources to provide services, and evaluation of services are other basic components of the system. It is only when all of these are brought together in a systematic process that involves the consumers, providers, and public officials of a health service area that it will be possible to specify the role that regulation should play in this system. To date, the regulatory process has evolved as though it were the only components of the system. The results have been particularly negative, as Harmon has so well documented.

Sixth, the role of the federal government in the new health planning system is confusing at this point. Harmon calls for greater intervention on the part of the federal government in delineating criteria and guidelines to specify what is expected of the states and regions in their regulatory functions. Although PL 93-641 is a beginning in this direction, the roles of the federal, state and local levels for carrying out planning and regulation are not clearly spelled out in the law. Because the de jure relationships are not made explicit in the law, the real relationships between the HSAs, health providers, and HEW planning agencies will be developed over time by the de facto linkages arising in day-to-day practices. Thus, while the law recognizes the need for the federal level to take a leadership role in fostering stronger regulatory controls, the same vagueness and ambiguity Harmon discovered in the existing system is still evident in the way the current law is written. There is more the appearance of a change in the law than a real one. The federal thrust is its threat to impose rigid, federally initiated regulations if the local and state planning agencies and the health providers do not work in a collaborative effort to affect cost control.

The Potential Impact of Federal Regulations on CON Review

In his analysis of what the federal regulations mean with respect to CON and 1122 criteria and procedures, Hanley makes it clear that the spirit of the law is toward an open, publicly involved democratic process. Access to almost all records not in violation of the privacy code; the posting of the time, place, and agenda of meetings; the publication and/or ready access by the public to reports, plans, and proposals subject to review before decisions are rendered; and encouraging the public to present verbal or written comments on any subject before the review body are some of the more significant features of the Act's procedures. This represents a considerable change as compared to the former, more secretive conduct of the planning agencies.

But, as significant as these procedural and participatory changes are in the Act, the criteria which all HSAs and SAs must adopt also are a departure from past practices. The federal government now states what the minimum criteria for reviewing a CON proposal must be. The Harmon study indicated that in the past, most agencies were very weak in their development and use of review criteria. However, what is lacking is specificity of what standards ought to be related to review criteria. For example, who determines and on what basis that a health provider has an adequate document for its long range plan? Who states when such a document is to be used as a criterion for review of a particular project? Who determines what the needs of a population in the community are and how those needs relate to the proposal submitted by the health provider? Thus, while there are statements in the law that serve as general guides for evaluating a CON proposal without standards, they are too vague in concept and too broad in scope to serve as meaningful criteria for review. The federal government appears willing at this time to permit local or state planning agencies to determine their own standards concerning the criteria. With this background, there are a number of implications for these procedures and criteria that require discussion.

First, the openness of the review process and the public's right to review the proposals can be expected to generate more competition and conflict than in the past. Health institutions expecting to propose services of a similar nature to the applicant, community leaders desiring influence in the affairs of the institution, or local political leaders seeking to score points with the community or the health provider all are in a position of making decisions in a glass bowl atmosphere. However, it can be anticipated that the novelty of contending over providers' proposals will wane, and decisions will be made more often than not in the relative calm of open meetings poorly attended by the public or its community leaders.

Second, the open process places pressure on the providers to develop complete, detailed proposals that specify objectives, target populations, costs, and impact on the existing medical system. This will represent a major change, as Harmon found that most CON proposals were poorly developed. In addition, this will require the provider to work more closely with the HSA staff, its board, and community leaders to win support for its proposals. Thus, in addition to better prepared proposals, one of the unanticipated consequences fostered by the Act will be the encouragement of closer relationships between health providers and community leaders located in subareas of the health service area.

Third, the HSA will be under pressure to develop precise definitions of its criteria and the standards that support them. This will have the advantageous effect of encouraging a more sophisticated HSA staff attuned to the nuances of the health system as well as adapting existing methods to create the standards needed to review various types of proposals. Thus, for example, a population's need for the proposed service could be defined from the point of view of a particular population, such as adolescents who live in inner cities or all adolescents in the entire region. It could be defined from the point of view of the medical institutions that serve these populations. Will it take into account the economic capacity of a population to pay for the services? Will it also include the capacity of the provider to offer services that cater to a population's linguistic (Spanish, Chinese, other) and religious values? The definition of need becomes far more complicated when such factors as these are linked to it. The difficulty of designing data systems and collecting the data that will permit planners to define need along one or more of these value dimensions may well set limits on how need is finally determined. But, it is more than need that requires definition and standards in the act's criteria. Alternative services, costs of service, manpower requirements, and an institution's long range plan all require definition before being used as quasi-scientific parameters for rendering decisions on CON proposals.

Fourth, and probably most important, a CON review decision must somehow or other be related to the Health Systems Plan and/or the Annual Implementation Plan. This carries with it other implications that deserve special attention.

The act is quite clear in specifying that a plan must be approved by the HSA and HEW before any review of CON can be undertaken. A virtual moratorium has thus been placed on the implementation of Title XVI and the authorization of funds under that act until both the State Health Plan and the State Medical Facilities Plan have been adopted. Likewise, the Health Development Fund will not be authorized for use until such plans are completed at the HSA level. This federal policy strongly implies that the state and regional plans are the primary means for determining the need for new institutional services, their expansion, or modernization. This means that review of CON and 1122 proposals will not be made in a vacuum as they have been in the past. The regulation function becomes a strategy for implementing the goals and objectives of the regional and state plans. By linking the two in this manner, the plans are no longer empty documents that gather dust on shelves. Consequently, the review of proposals will be made on a more rational basis that should stand the test of community need. The rationality of the process does not mean that CON reviews are divorced from social and political influence. It means that a standard (the HSP and the AIP) which has survived political and social pressures, including public scrutiny and comment, will have been developed and will have provided a community basis for decisionmaking. Such decisions will no longer be made on a case-by-case basis.

However, if planning becomes inextricably joined to the regulatory function, the question is whether or not they can live compatibly under the same HSA roof? Several critics have indicated that the characteristics of the two functions are so diverse, and possibly in conflict with each other, that they should be separated, with the state assuming the regulatory function and the HSA the planning function. These critics point out that the state already has been granted de jure authority to make the final decision on CON and 1122 proposals. Why not give them complete de facto power to deal with the entire function? The fact of the matter is that although the HSAs have only de facto power over such proposals (they can only recommend approval or disapproval to the state agency), these advisory decisions carry considerable weight and are more often than not accepted by the state agency on the premise that the HSAs know best what is needed for their areas.

Perhaps an examination of these two important functions is in order. Chapter one alluded to the planning function as dynamic, evolving, comprehensive, responsive to local social, economic and cultural values, normative in the decisions that are made, future oriented, and responsive to the latest in technological or medical delivery trends. The regulatory function, in contrast, is rigid, routinized, narrow as to how proposals are reviewed, responsive primarily to technical and other accepted criteria, bureaucratic in the way decisions are ultimately made, present oriented in that the concern is for how the project will meet current rather than future needs, and usually inimical to the latest technological or delivery system trends. The plan is a political document based on community consensus, while the review decision is a legal decision based on authority mandated by legislation or regulations.

Because the priorities of a plan are expected to change in response to technological changes or shifts in population, the basis for determining a community's need for services will also change. Can it be expected that the rigid criteria and standards used in the regulatory function will permit flexibility and change? If not, it may well be that the regulatory staff will be approving expansion of HMOs in a community based on the old plan's priorities when, in fact, a trend toward home-based and mobile services may have supplanted HMOs as the higher priority. Without close coordination and a capacity for the regulatory arm of the HSA to be responsive to the planning function, tensions will be created between the two. Because a plan's goals are but one basis for determining which CON proposals to approve or disapprove, the regulatory arm may well use its legal authority to march to one drummer while the rest of the HSA marches to another. Yet, different as these two sets of characteristics are, there are experts who agree they can be carried out under the same HSA roof if the plan is indeed comprehensive, detailed, and specific, and if the staff and board work together.

While a plan may offer a basis for evaluating the need of a single proposal, it offers little guidance as to how to deal with competing applications, both of which meet the plan's goal requirements, criteria, and other technical standards of the review process. How does one select? Who should do the choosing? What are the implications of the HSA's choosing one applicant over another? And what if the plan does not address itself to proposals requesting CONs? Are the reviews made without consideration of the future needs of such services in the region? Are the reviews made with review staff only, or with collaboration of the planning staff? If amendments to the plan result in drastic changes of priorities for the region, should the review staff take these changes into account in making its decision? What was acceptable last year may no longer be approvable this year. How does one respond to providers who have been preparing proposals at some cost to themselves based on the old priorities of the plan? These are thorny questions which require guidance for the health providers. As will be noted below, failure to provide such direction may well lead to a number of appeals and/or legal suits. Thus, while the linkage of regulation to planning represents a step forward, it raises other issues formerly of little concern to the planning agencies that require solutions.

There is, in addition, another question that can be raised about the relationship between the planning and regulatory function. While planning does add a positive link to the review process, it also creates complications if the two opposing characteristics and roles are not firmly kept in mind. Up to now, the regulatory function has received the primary attention of comprehensive health planning agencies. For the first year or two of the HSA's existence, the planning function will be given primary consideration. However, when the review process begins in earnest, which will become the dominant activity the HSA? If the continued emphasis on cost containment over the meeting of local health service needs remains the dominant issue, then obviously the regulatory function will be paramount. More likely, a balance will be found between the two where planning will be the guiding force in the decisionmaking and the implementation of programs under CON and 1122 reviews. Yet, because the characteristics of the two functions are so different, it can be anticipated that these differences may be a considerable source of conflict within the

HSA as attempts are made to allocate resources, staff, and board time to their respective functions.

Legal Threats to CON Review

Glantz has classified a number of actual and potential challenges to the CON laws. He points out that with the exception of North Carolina's overturning of its CON law, none of the challenges in other states has posed any real danger to CON laws. However, based on the decision of the North Carolina supreme court to rule the CON law unconstitutional, a further court suit has been brought by that state against the United States. The essential complaint is that the United States Congress is interfering with North Carolina's right to govern its state by requiring it to pass a CON law (which it has previously declared unconstitutional) in order to receive federal grants needed to maintain the health and safety of its citizens. This suit represents a major attack on the legitimacy of an important function of PL 93-641—its requirement that all states carry out review functions under Section 1513—and could well endanger the entire system of planning, regulation, and implementation embodied in the law.

If this aspect of the law is found unconstitutional, then a reversion to the situation prior to the passage of the law would exist. All of the arguments and evidence previously cited concerning the weakness and ineffectiveness of CON laws would prevail, severely undermining the cost containment policy of the federal government. Further, it would damage the necessary link between planning and regulation previously discussed so that each would be done (or not done) independently of the other. All of the problems noted in previous sections of this chapter and in other chapters of this book would continue. This challenge to the law thus represents a most serious threat to both the CON review process and the effectiveness of the Act itself.

In addition to this challenge, there are two other legal issues with important implications for CON review. The first refers to the handling of competing applications where a regional plan has been adopted. Under such circumstances, Glantz points out that where two or more applicants are equally capable of providing the services called for in the HSP, a review of one such health provider's proposal cannot be made until the other providers have an opportunity to present their proposals.

The time period for preparing, reviewing, appealing, and implementing a health provider's proposal would be considerably increased and might well affect HSA or state review schedules. The Act now calls for a maximum of 90 days for the entire review process. (Additional time is permitted for appeals.) However, how is this process to be completed within the 90-day period if applicant A must wait the submission of applicant B or C's proposal so they can be reviewed simultaneously? Because applicants B and C already have access to A's proposal, they are in a position to improve upon any perceived weaknesses in that proposal while developing their own. How fair is this to applicant A, and does the 90-day review period for applicant A start upon the notification of the receipt of its applications by the HSA as the law requires? If so, and the proposals of applicants B and C take another 30 days to submit, how can they be reviewed simultaneously when each of their review periods starts at different times? The HSA can well be challenged by applicant A for not providing "due process" to all the applicants. To avoid this allegation, the HSA will have to prepare guidelines for dealing with multiple competing applications.

The second implication refers to how decisions are made on competing applications when all health providers appear to have adequate competency to achieve the goals of the HSP. The HSA has to develop standards in advance of engaging in the review function. This can be accomplished in collaboration with health providers and considered part of its review procedures as required under Section 1532 of PL 93-641. Otherwise, a disapproved health provider may be in a position to challenge the HSA's decision on the basis of arbitrariness and unfairness even though the HSA may have made the best decision. While difficult, with the assistance of providers and prior experience in CON reviews, most HSAs are capable of setting such standards.

The third implication resulting from rendering decisions on competing applications is that the stage is set for developing the very conflicts and adversary relationships that are detrimental to the development and implementation of the plan's goals. It is the providers in the health service areas that must implement the goals. Their collaboration and good will are essential if this is to occur. If the unsuccessful provider refuses to collaborate with the HSA in future situations requiring its involvement, then that segment of the delivery system will have broken down. To avoid such confrontations, some critics of CON laws have strongly recommended that the HSAs merely testify as to whether the competing applications meet their minimum standards or not. Then, they suggest that the final decision be made by the state agency, which already has this obligation and authority by law. This would have the effect of preserving the tenuous, fragile local relationships among the providers while permitting the state agency to render a more objective decision since it is not involved on a daily basis with the competing applicants.

The second legal issue which requires some discussion refers to the potential illegality of planning agencies to set conditions on health provider proposals before having them approved. Hanley has suggested in his chapter that this is a tactic which is currently used to discourage applicants from applying for CONs or to condition the approval on the willingness of the provider to amend the proposal to meet the objectives of the HSA. There is little question but that a number of situations will be arising in which the HSA risks influencing a health provider rather than evaluating his proposal on its merits and according to the criteria previously defined in its published procedures manual. To avoid litigation that could easily arise in these circumstances, the HSA and the health providers must work together so that each knows what to expect of the other and can assist the other in meeting mutual needs. While there are other legal implications that will arise from the implementation of PL 93-641, those discussed above are more conspicuous and call for HSA and provider collaboration and resolution.

Methods for Developing Plans and Proposals

There are two interesting conclusions that Crane draws in his chapter on methodology. The first is that while there are a number of methods for forecasting future medical facility needs, all of these, except the stochastic method, provide projections at the regional rather than the institutional level of planning. Yet, one of the limitations of the stochastic method is its inability to project future population or institutional need. The second conclusion is that no one method by itself has the capacity to forecast both need and demand. According to Crane, "some combination of these or other methods will most likely serve to fit a particular user's needs." Thus, no one way has yet been discovered that can be routinely applied for determining a community's or an institution's future need. Crane's major contribution has been to the major methods now in use, identifying their strengths and limitations and relating them to both the planning process and the criteria required by the act. What do these findings mean for HSAs and health providers?

While there is enough known about the application of methods for HSAs to begin work on their plans, much research is required to test the efficacy of these various methods and to find the best means to forecast future need. For example, the Hill-Burton formulas in conjunction with population surveys such as those conducted in Rhode Island can describe a more realistic picture of need than can the Hill-Burton formula alone.

Once need is identified, a number of different alternative strategies may be developed to meet those needs. This will involve the cooperative efforts of the health providers because they know first-hand the probable cost and staffing requirements in the use of one medical service versus another. In the Thompson case illustration Medeiros pointed out that the surplus beds in that health service area could easily be used by the providers to meet other population health problems such as those related to mental illness, alcoholism, and day care needs that were not being met. Through the collaborative efforts of the HSAs and the health providers, the meeting of needs becomes both a technical and a normative process. While the potential for conflict exists between the two parties, the rewards will come from making decisions as to how best to use resources currently available.

The final implication is that although there is no mechanical, "canned" method for developing institutional proposals, there is much guidance in the form of HSPs and their goals, criteria, and procedures manuals to assist the health providers in developing proposals that are consistent with the goals of the HSP and their own institutions. The HSAs are also in a position to supply the provider with the data to determine the need for the service or facility, to clarify and interpret what criteria are applicable, and to provide technical assistance in developing the proposal. Through this collaborative process, sound proposals can be arrived at by health providers to meet the high priority objectives of the HSP.

ACTIONS FOR HEALTH PROVIDER CONSIDERATION

The central thrusts of PL 93-641 have changed the nature of the planning-regulatory-resources systems. In the past, the system was divided into three parallel systems, each autonomous (the planning system of the CHPs, the regulatory system of the states and Hill-Burton agencies, and the resources system of federal grants and RMP funding). All these systems were reactive in that the health provider made requests or sought out certificates or fundings, and the system reacted to those requests in a positive, negative, or ambiguous manner. The integration of these three systems as subsystems of the health planning and resources development system has drastically changed the role and status of the actors. It is no longer possible for a health provider to ignore the other two systems. Planning is not separate from regulation or implementation. Therefore, the provider must take all three subsystems into account before dealing with any one part of the system. If, for example, the provider wants to add an emergency service to his facility, he must find out whether the

HSP requires such an emergency service. He must find out whether the resources that are normally available for such services will be allocated to his institution, or whether they are being considered for an alternative way of delivering those services? While it may be possible for one part of the health planning system not to know what the other parts are engaged in, this is less likely to occur in an organizationally integrated system than in separate and autonomous systems. Further, it is far easier to identify and resolve problems within one system than in separate systems. Thus, while the new health planning law does not add anything really new to the previous three separate planning systems, this is a case where the new system as a whole is greater than the sum of its parts.

The fact that the health provider must keep in mind the system as a whole also radically changes his role in relation to that system. Through the development of an HSP, review criteria, procedures, and standards, the HSA becomes the initiator of what it expects from the health provider and not the other way around. This requires a major mental shift, and it will take some time and experience before the health providers learn to adjust. How the health providers react to this shift will determine the future relationship between the HSA and the providers.

In spite of the two major shifts in the health planning field noted above, the central fact continues to be that the health provider is the agent that can make or break the planning-regulatory-implementation system. As autonomous actors in a complicated delivery system, they must choose to work or not to work with the HSA. Regardless of what the HSA proposes, the health providers as independent actors cannot be forced into doing anything that is contrary to their institutional interests. This independent stance can be maintained only as long as the health provider does not have to come to the HSA for its approval of a CON, a federal grant, demonstration grants or technical assistance. However, since it is inconceivable that a health provider can indefinitely maintain his "business as usual" operation in this day of rapid technological, legislative, regulatory, and administrative changes, at some point he will have to touch base with the HSA. The question is, how can the provider best relate to the HSA given this change in the HSA's power and its role as leader and initiator in the health planning-regulatory system. The recommended actions described below are based on the assumption that the initial relationship between the two parties will be fraught with conflict, as Medeiros asserts in his chapter. But, over time, new, more stable relationships will be formed between the HSA and the provider institutions.

This evolving change in relationships and attitudes has nowhere been better demonstrated than in the Rochester, New York area. There providers were involved in formulating the initial plans and standards for acute care facilities. The first efforts at implementation of those plans and the many disapprovals that flowed from the fact of over-bedding led to much disgruntlement on the part of providers. Their appeals to the political and economic decision-makers in the community went unheeded because they were made conscious of the cost of unused beds and services to the region. While exceptions were considered, as in the Thompson case, the rule was to disapprove and seek alternative, less costly methods for providing the services, if need could be demonstrated. In time, the providers have come to accept that the plan and its standards are documents that guide what will be accomplished in the region. While there are confrontations that occasionally erupt, for the most part the health providers are learning to live with and use the plan for providing services that are needed for the various target populations, and at lower costs to the community and taxpayers. The concept of planning-regulation-implementation is working in one community. It can work elsewhere.

What are some of the actions health providers can take in this newly developing situation? The first function that is being stressed by HSAs and SAs is the planning function. And the component of planning that will be receiving major attention will be health facilities, particularly acute care and long term nursing home facilities. Since the law mandates that one-third of the providers on the HSA governing body must be physicians and hospital administrators from among direct providers, it can be assumed that their point of view on the health plan concerned with health facilities will be well represented. The first action these provider governing body members should take is to chair and be represented on those committees and task forces responsible for developing the acute care and nursing home components of the HSP. Past experience indicates that they will influence the consumer and public official members of the committees to accept their point of view. The challenge to the committees' recommendations will come when they compete with other committees and their representatives concerned with other facets of health such as health education, environmental health problems, HMOs, and mental health. In the arena of competing interests they should, however, be in a position to wield substantial influence in achieving acceptance of a number of their concerns as high-priority goals.

In the process of developing the HSP, the HSA is going to require data from many different sources in order to set goals and make decisions based on facts. Individual health providers have an abundance of data to offer the HSAs such as utilization rates, demographic facts on its clientele, manpower ratios, and cost of operating its various services. By sharing such data with the HSAs, the health providers would be in a position in the future to use the aggregated data to develop their own proposals. Not only would they have their own data, but also that of other institutions. To be sure, sharing data means that the individual health providers expose themselves to inspection by the public as well as by their competitors. The data can be used to criticize them as well as to support them. If some of the criticism is valid, then it will serve to prod them into improving themselves, and it will also lead to the community's needs being served in a more efficient and effective manner. The provider, in turn, can offer valid criticism of the proposals of other health institutions. The reciprocal and collective scrutiny that the HSA, the public, and providers give to CON proposals can, therefore, produce long run positive improvement in the health delivery system. The price of having to endure short run criticism by sharing data and opening up to public evaluation is minor compared to the long run benefits for all.

Many health providers, particularly hospitals, are members of associations which work in their common interests. While these associations do protect and promote the positive image of its members to the public, they may also cover up the limited ways that hospitals and other providers actually work together to foster a more efficient and effective delivery system. This was especially noticed in the Thompson case where Medeiros cited how the hospitals in the region were not ready to decertify even two beds to assist the needs of the Thompson Hospital, even though the region was overbedded by 60 or more. It seems that integrated and coordinated planning mandated by the national goals of PL 93-641 require a new working arrangement among the health providers. Individual institutional needs must be blended with those of community needs that are articulated in the goals and priorities of the HSP. This will require the providers either to redirect the orientation of their existing professional associations or to create new consortia for the purpose of allocating resources and providing services within the constraints of the HSP's goals. While differences will emerge, they do not have to degenerate into adversary or conflicting relationships. The providers can, with some compromise and acceptance of the changed nature of their role as autonomous agents within a structured delivery system, give up some of their individual autonomy for the common good. The consortium is the place where they can work out these new relationships and have them incorporated into various aspects of the HSP concerned with hospital facilities and services. The consortium would have many influential, natural allies on the HSA's governing body and its various committees who would be expected to be sympathetic to the interests of the consortium. Indeed, if the members could work out their own relationships within the structure of the consortium, they would be in a positive position to provide much of the planning expertise for the HSA as it relates to their interests.

As has been said previously, the health providers are the key actors in the implementation of HSA goals and the primary recipients of resources allocated under PL 93-641 and federal agencies for providing services to the community. However, because of the review functions mandated to HSAs under PL 93-641, in particular the regulatory function of CON and 1122 reviews, the demonstration of prospective rate review systems being carried out in half a dozen states, the reviews required of proposals for federally funded projects under both Titles XV and XVI of PL 93-641, and the periodic reviews of all existing health facilities and services as to their appropriateness, the course these reviews take and the policies and new federal, state and local initiatives which may follow pose both opportunities and dangers to the health providers and the way they currently deliver services. To insure that their interests receive a fair hearing with respect to these various reviews, the health providers should volunteer their services to assist the HSAs in such tasks as the development of standards for determining appropriateness of quality and quantity of services, and development of guidelines that will encourage experiments and innovations in the provision of services or alternative delivery mechanisms. By their involvement in such activities, the health providers will be in a position to reduce the adversary nature of their roles with respect to the HSA and to replace it with a more permissive and collaborative one. Through this type of relationship, the number of legal challenges to the HSA can also be mitigated. Thus, while the providers will not be able to prevent the various regulating functions from taking place, their active involvement at the very outset on the process will permit them to influence the direction and potential impact on their institutions.

In recent years, the development of computer sciences and esoteric statistical and mathematical concepts has increasingly found the decision-makers in the health field dependent on technocrats who control these new analytical techniques. In the process, they have given up some of their decisionmaking function to these technocrats. Among these technocrats are the planners, statisticians, fiscal experts, architects, and systems analysts. All of these experts are essential in providing the technical background material and in identifying alternatives upon which the decision-makers can make their choices. It is up to the health providers (physicians, nurses, hospital administrators, trustees) to work with consumers and public officials to prevent the technocrats from asserting their dominance in decisionmaking based solely on technical considerations. As Medeiros has pointed out, there are a number of normative values (social, cultural, economic) on which decisions can also be based. Only the natural leaders and decision-makers in the health field are in a position to add these other criteria to the technical considerations in making decisions. By doing so, the decision-makers, including the influential health providers, are in a position to demonstrate their accountability and concern to all segments of the population. They are in a position to think through the alternatives and the policies implied in them. In asserting themselves in their role as decision-makers (whether formal members of the HSA governing body or one of its committees, as representatives of health provider consortia who can informally make known their views) they place the technocrats in their proper role as servants of the governing body even while permitting them to have a voice in the deliberations on the basis of their knowledge. Health providers are particularly comfortable in dealing with the technocrats of their own institutions and, as such, would be in a position of reasserting this relationship in the context of the HSA's decisionmaking structure.

While there are other actions that health providers can engage in, those discussed above should highlight the direction these actions might take. They have an important role to play in the new HSA. That role can be one of acting as an adversary or as a collaborator. In either instance, they encounter much difficulty in working with the HSA in the establishment of the new planning system and their acceptance of the regulatory function. This requires an altered way of thinking and a new maturity in order to transfer from autonomous entrepreneurs in a fragmented system to working in concert with other parts of the delivery system to help it become an integrated, efficient, and effective system that serves the entire community as well as the interests of the institutions. That is the goal of PL 93-641, and that should be the goal of those involved in the delivery of medical services.

About the Author

Herbert H. Hyman, Ph.D., is Associate Professor of Urban Affairs, Hunter College. He recently served as a consultant to the Bureau of Health Planning in the Department of Health, Education and Welfare.

Dr. Hyman is a noted authority in the fields of urban and health planning. He received the Superior Performance Award from the Veterans Administration in 1964 and was the first "Social Worker of the Year" to be chosen by the National Association of Social Workers, Connecticut Chapter. Dr. Hyman was awarded the NASPPA Fellowship for 1975-1976. Other books by Dr. Hyman include, *The Politics of Health Planning* and *Health Planning: A Systematic Approach.*